I0479307

DISRUPTIVE MOOD DYSREGULATION DISORDER

An Empowering Integrative Guide for Parents

COPYRIGHT © 2023, by Scott A. Johnson

All Rights Reserved. No part of this publication may be reproduced or transmitted in any form or by any means, electronic or mechanical, including photocopying and recording, or introduced into any information storage and retrieval system without the written permission of the copyright owner. Brief quotations may be used in reviews prepared for magazines, blogs, newspapers, or broadcasts.

Disruptive Mood Dysregulation Disorder: An Empowering Integrative Guide for Parents / Scott A. Johnson

Cover design: Scott A. Johnson

Cover Copyright: © Scott A. Johnson 2023

ISBN-13: 979-8376881347

Discover more books by Scott A. Johnson at authorscott.com.

Published by Scott A. Johnson Professional Writing Services, LLC: Orem, UT

DISCLAIMERS OF WARRANTY AND LIMITATION OF LIABILITY

The author provides all information on an "as is" and "as available" basis and for informational purposes only. The author makes no representations or warranties of any kind, expressed or implied, as to the information, materials, or products mentioned. Every effort has been made to ensure accuracy and completeness of the information contained; however, it is not intended to replace any medical advice or to halt proper medical treatment, nor diagnose, treat, cure, or prevent any health condition or disease.

Always consult a qualified medical professional before using any dietary supplement or natural product, engaging in physical activity, or modifying your diet; and seek the advice of your physician with any questions you may have regarding any medical condition. Always consult your OB/GYN if you are pregnant or think you may become pregnant before using any dietary supplement or natural product, and to ensure you are healthy enough for exercise or any dietary modifications. The information contained in this book is for educational and informational purposes only, and it is not meant to replace medical advice, diagnosis, or treatment in any manner. Never delay or disregard professional medical advice. Use the information solely at your own risk; the author accepts no responsibility for the use thereof. This book is sold with the understanding that neither the author nor publisher shall be liable for any loss, injury, or harm allegedly arising from any information or suggestion in this book.

The Food and Drug Administration (FDA) has not evaluated the statements contained in this book. The information and materials are not meant to diagnose, prescribe, or treat any disease, condition, illness, or injury. You are encouraged to seek the most current information and medical care from your healthcare professional.

To exhausted parents who through tear-filled eyes, earnest prayers, and great anxiety seek answers to help their precious child feel better and realize his or her gull potential. May this book provide greater understanding, comfort, and hope.

Contents

1

....

AN INTRODUCTION TO DISRUPTIVE MOOD DYSREGULATION DISORDER

Modern society has fueled a pediatric mental health crisis with an alarming number of children and teens experiencing anxiety, depression, and other mood disorders. This crisis has become so severe that in 2021 the American Academy of Pediatrics along with the American Academy of Child Adolescent Psychiatry and the Children's Hospital Association declared child and adolescent health a national emergency.[1] In this declaration, these organizations pleaded for increased funding for mental health resources, better integration of mental health care in schools and primary care, additional community resources, more mental health professionals, and better insurance coverage for mental health care. These are each necessary to combat this crisis affecting our children, but most important is to equip you, the parents, with vital information and effective tools to help guide your children through this predicament.

Another hurdle to overcome to improve our gigantic pediatric mental health crisis is to reduce the stigma of mental illness. A stigma is when someone views another person in a negative way because of a distinguishing characteristic or trait that society believes is a disadvantage. Although we have come a long way from sequestering the mentally ill in insane asylums and have gained a far greater understanding of mental health and behavioral disorders in recent years, we nevertheless have a long way to go. For far too long, people with mental illnesses have been told to suck it up, try harder, improve their character or willpower, or simply get over it. Imagine telling a person with diabetes, arthritis, or another physical illness to simply get over it and suck it up. This would be unfathomable, yet it is commonly told to people with genuine mental health or mood disorders.

In its place, we need to show greater compassion and be more mindful of other people's emotions. People who suffer from mental illness and associated behavioral and neurological disorders must often build walls and play a part, a façade, if you will, so that others will not notice that they are experiencing negative emotions at the time. This is incredibly draining and invalidating to these courageous individuals. A solid first step is the mere acknowledgement that someone else is struggling and showing them that you care. Recognize that their situation is difficult and challenging, and then verbalize this understanding to them. It can be as straightforward as stating, "I'm sorry you are going through this. It sounds difficult. I'm so glad you shared with me, and I am here to listen. What can I do to help you?" We must tear down the labelling, stereotyping, and discrimination that gives power to stigma against mental illness for these brave individuals to receive the support they need in a future of ever-increasing mental and emotional disorders.

A relatively new—first appearing in the Diagnostic and Statistical Manual of Mental Disorders, Fifth Edition (DSM-

5) in 2013[2]—and underrecognized mood disorder is disruptive mood dysregulation disorder (DMDD). DMDD is a condition in children, adolescents, and teens characterized by ongoing irritability, anger, and frequent, intense temper outbursts. While youth can get depressed or feel discouraged or a sense of hopelessness, DMDD is more than a "bad mood"; the chronic irritability leads to unrelenting eruptions of severe anger and recurrent temper tantrums. Children with DMDD experience emotions on a much stronger level than their peers and more frequently feel irritability, anger, and other negative emotions. Small matters significantly irritate them, and these stronger emotions can quickly overwhelm them, triggering verbal or physical aggression. If the immediate environment they are in does not meet their demands, they further destabilize.

Furthermore, your child struggles to correctly identify and label his own emotions, which decreases social awareness and the ability to recognize the emotions of those around him. These deficits make him lack empathy for others and struggle to regulate his emotions. For example, instead of defaulting to anger over a sibling or friend's action, a neurotypical adolescent or teen will consider the circumstances that led to the action, possible reasons for the action, and appropriate responses to maintain a healthy relationship. Instead, your child with DMDD takes the action personally and feels the need to respond aggressively. Sometimes he'll even retaliate and feel the need to "get even." Due to insufficient empathy, he may also do things that irritate others because he doesn't recognize his actions are bothering those around him. For instance, he may play his music very loudly because he enjoys it, not understanding that he is disrupting his older sister's homework. The hazards of poor emotional regulation are anxiety, fear, anger, overreaction, and harm to relationships.

DMDD is typically diagnosed by age ten and affects youth between the ages of two and seventeen (although diagnosis cannot be official until at least six years old), with the highest occurrence in preschool-age children.[3] It is estimated that the condition affects between 0.8 percent and 3.3 percent of children aged two to seventeen, and as high as 8.2 percent in six-year-olds.[4,5] Because it is a relatively new diagnosis, its prevalence is likely significantly underestimated. Indeed, the symptom profile of DMDD appears in youths at an astonishing rate of 26 to 31 percent.[6] It is more commonly diagnosed among boys than girls. Overall, symptoms affect your child's quality of life and relationships at home and school and among friends.

Although symptoms—like temper tantrums and irritability—usually decrease as the child transitions to young adulthood, living in the midst of this tumultuous time until adulthood is very trying for the child, his siblings, parents, teachers, and peers. The reality is that symptoms don't just disappear once your child reaches adulthood. They don't grow out of it with age. Instead, doctors begin to consider another mental health or mood disorder is to blame for the symptoms as your child reaches adulthood. This may be primarily due to the diagnostics criteria that disallow diagnosis of DMDD after age seventeen. Indeed, DMDD was introduced as a mood disorder because few children with chronic mood disorders progressed to develop adult bipolar affective disorder.[7] Youth with DMDD may experience trouble in school and have difficulty maintaining healthy connections and relationships with family members or peers. They have a hard time finding their people and tribe due to deep-seated trust issues. Social settings and team activities may also be challenging. Regrettably, DMDD frequently transitions to depression or anxiety as the child develops.

Manifesting as persistent and extreme irritability and anger, DMDD is distinguished from other mood disorders by frequent, developmentally inappropriate temper outbursts involving rages of verbal or physically aggressive behavior toward people or property. The DMDD diagnostics criteria were established to more accurately diagnose youth who may have previously been diagnosed with pediatric bipolar disorder despite not meeting the full criteria for this diagnosis. The DMDD diagnosis resulted from a previously diagnosed subtype of bipolar disorder called severe mood dysregulation disorder (SMD). Symptoms of DMDD may also overlap with, or occur at the same time (comorbid) as, attention deficit hyperactivity disorder (ADHD; nearly all youth with DMDD have ADHD as well; comorbidity 86.9%–93.8%), oppositional defiant disorder (ODD; comorbidity 84.4%–84.9%), and anxiety (comorbidity 46.9%–58.2%).[8,9] This makes an accurate diagnosis and identification of comorbidities essential to formulate an effective treatment plan. To avoid the use of multiple medications required to address specific symptoms, some experts suggest therapeutic intervention should be focused on treating the comorbid disorder instead.

To learn more about ADHD and natural solutions to manage it, refer to this author's book *Beating ADHD Naturally*.

Differentiating DMDD and Adolescent Bipolar Disorder

BIPOLAR	DMDD
Develops during late adolescence or early adulthood	Develops earlier and only diagnosed between 6–18 years
Manic or hypomanic episodes	Manic/hypomanic episodes absent
Extreme irritation only occurs during manic episodes	Irritation and anger occur are persistent between outbursts
Psychotic symptoms may be observed	Absence of psychotic symptoms
Parental history of bipolar disorder	Usually, no parental history of bipolar disorder

The DSM-5 includes the following as criteria for diagnosing DMDD:

A. Severe recurrent temper outbursts manifested verbally and/or behaviorally that are grossly out of proportion in intensity or duration to the situation or provocation.

B. Temper outbursts are inconsistent with developmental level.

C. Temper outbursts occur, on average, three or more times per week.

D. Mood between temper outbursts is persistently irritable or angry most of the day, nearly every day, and is observable by others.

E. Criteria A–D have been present for one year or longer without a lapse in any of the symptoms lasting three or more consecutive months.

F. Criteria A–D are present in at least two of the following settings: home, school, with peers; and are severe in at least one.

G. Diagnosis should not be made for the first time before age six or after age eighteen.

H. The age of onset of criteria A–E is before ten years.

I. There has never been a distinct period lasting more than one day during which the full symptom criteria, except duration, for a manic or hypomanic episode have been met.

J. The behaviors do not occur exclusively during an episode of major depressive disorder and are not better explained by another mental disorder (e.g., autism, PTSD, anxiety, or persistent depressive disorder).

K. The symptoms are not attributable to the physiological effects of a substance or to another medical or neurological condition.

Although currently categorized as a depressive disorder, new evidence suggests it may be better categorized as a behavioral disorder. Specifically, a longitudinal study found that 96 percent of youth with DMDD also met criteria for the behavioral disorders ODD and conduct disorder (CD); while 77 percent met criteria for an ADHD and ODD/CD diagnosis.[10] This emphasizes the importance of identifying any comorbidities with DMDD, especially since substance abuse may indicate self-medicating of a mood disorder, and a history of trauma is linked to mood disorders, CD, substance abuse, and disruptive symptoms.

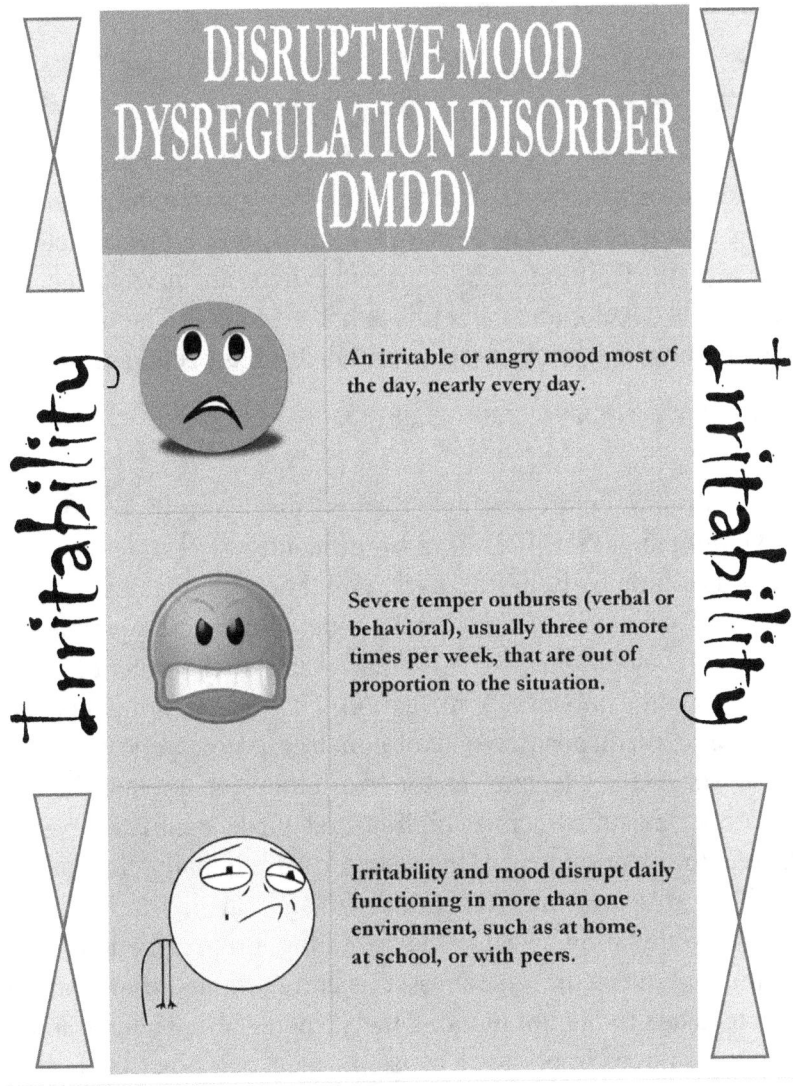

DISRUPTIVE MOOD DYSREGULATION DISORDER (DMDD)

An irritable or angry mood most of the day, nearly every day.

Severe temper outbursts (verbal or behavioral), usually three or more times per week, that are out of proportion to the situation.

Irritability and mood disrupt daily functioning in more than one environment, such as at home, at school, or with peers.

Irritability

Irritability

Youth with DMDD are at an increased risk of poverty, violent relationships, STIs (sexually transmitted infections), substance abuse, suspension from school, and engaging in risky behaviors. This is to be expected when they unsuccessfully learned social and emotional cues that gradually teach children appropriate and expected responses in society. Although parents should keep these problems in mind, it doesn't mean your child is doomed to an awful future. Proper intervention can mitigate some of these potential negative outcomes.

CAUSES

The exact cause of DMDD is not known, but like most other mood disorders, it is likely caused by a combination of environmental, biological, psychological, and genetic factors. We are still learning and discovering more about what factors lead to its development and this is hotly debated. The one thing we do know is that no single causal factor has been identified.

ENVIRONMENTAL FACTORS

One of the environmental factors that contribute to the development of DMDD is a significantly stressful event or period of time early in life. Early childhood trauma (emotional, physical, or sexual) is linked to the development and aggravation of DMDD symptoms.[11,12,13] It could occur after a recent family death, divorce, job loss, or relocation. The current thought is that a genetic predisposition—serotonin transporter gene, FKBP5 gene, or other genetic factor—to mood or mental health disorders exists in some children and these traumatic events trigger the development of the disorder.[14] Essentially, the trauma initiates structural and functional changes in the brain, alters DNA methylation (further deteriorating brain function over time), and interferes with stress axis and immune-inflammatory mechanisms to disrupt mood. Other experts believe that trauma history is not as important a causal influence as other factors.

A lack of adequate nutrition is also a factor, and science has found that poor nutrition during the first few years of life can lead to antisocial, aggressive, and other behavioral problems later in childhood.[15] Poor nutritional choices deprive the body of nutrients vital for neurological development such as protein, zinc, iron, and B vitamins. Several studies have shown that deficiencies in B vitamins—niacin, pantothenic acid, thiamin, B6—and vitamin C are associated with irritability.[16,17,18,19,20] B vitamins can be found in watermelon, whole grains, legumes, bananas, eggs, and dairy products. Vitamin D deficiency is associated with depression and aggressive and rule-breaking behaviors.[21,22] It is very difficult to get enough vitamin D from food alone, but it is found in fish, egg yolks, and mushrooms. Iron is critical for dopamine neurotransmission, and insufficient amounts of iron can cause learning deficits and behavioral problems.[23,24] Red meat is usually the primary source of iron. It is also obtained from poultry, eggs, and green vegetables. Magnesium plays a crucial role in regulating neurotransmitter balance and affects one's ability to cope with stress, which could contribute to abnormal behaviors.[25,26] Spinach, broccoli, seeds, and legumes are all good sources of magnesium. The essential amino acid tryptophan, a component of protein, is necessary in the diet to produce serotonin. Serotonin is a major neurotransmitter and decreased levels are associated with aggressive, violent, impulsive, and suicidal behavior.[27,28] Poultry, salmon, tuna, and edamame are good food sources of tryptophan. It is possible that overaggressive behavior, irritability, and mood are a manifestation of an underlying nutrient deficiency or insufficiency due to poor nutrition. The best way to overcome this is obviously to improve your child's diet, but even the best child or youth diet will benefit from smart supplementation of key or deficient/insufficient nutrients.

Mental health and mood disorders may also be related to food allergies or sensitivities.[29] To better understand the connection between food sensitivity and these disorders, we need to discuss the gut-brain axis. This term describes the two-way communication that occurs between the gastrointestinal tract (gut) and the brain. The gut sends signals to the brain, which in turn influences nervous system responses and the brain sends signals to the gut influencing gut function. This communication channel is controlled by the immune, endocrine, and central nervous systems, which are all influenced by the bacteria present in the gut (gut microbiome). The diversity and quantity of bacteria in the gut microbiome directly impact one's susceptibility to food sensitivities and intolerance. The lining of your child's digestive tract provides a barrier between what is consumed and the rest of the body. Poor integrity of these linings, called leaky gut, can allow pathogens, toxins, and large food molecules to exit the gut and enter the bloodstream that shouldn't be there. These foreign invaders in the bloodstream are detected by the immune system, which mounts a response that is controlled by immunoglobulin G (IgG). Food intolerances or sensitivities are mediated by IgG antibodies and can take up to forty-eight hours to have an effect. With poor gut integrity and an unhealthy gut microbiome, the immune system is overwhelmed, and its response is persistent. Chronic immune responses can negatively impact the brain and its function leading to mood and mental health issues.[30] The term *nervous stomach* may actually be grounded in neuroscience because poor gut health can trigger anxiety, depression, and other mood problems.

An out-of-balance brain can cause digestive system dysfunction, which further causes the immune system to get out of balance. Conversely, a food sensitivity can trigger an immune system reaction that instigates an immune system response flooding the body with inflammatory cytokines. Cytokines can inflame the gut, brain, joint, or respiratory tract and alter the way your child feels physically, mentally, and emotionally. Ultimately, this leads to food sensitivities. Common food intolerances include dairy, eggs, gluten (a protein found in wheat, rye, oats, and barley), sugar (especially if *Candida* overgrowth is present), soy, shellfish, high salicylate foods, food dyes, preservatives, genetically modified foods (GMOs), herbicides (glyphosate being chief among them), and pesticides. Food allergies/sensitivities could be a contributing factor to many mental-health-related or behavioral issues, including DMDD.

REACTIVE HYPOGLYCEMIA

Reactive hypoglycemia (RH; also called postprandial hypoglycemia or sugar crash) refers to the occurrence of low blood sugar after eating—usually two to four hours later. It is characterized by hunger, irritability, weakness, shakiness, paleness, lightheadedness, moodiness, anxiety, behavioral changes (tantrums, sudden crying without a reason), sugar cravings, nightmares, confusion on waking, and sweating. While the exact cause of RH is unknown, it may be the result of the pancreas making too much insulin, particularly after a large, carb-heavy meal. Essentially, the pancreas continues to secrete insulin despite the glucose from the meal being handled. The extra insulin in the bloodstream decreases blood sugar levels to below normal, triggering the release of stress hormones to stimulate the replenishment of blood sugar from internal and external (food, drink) sources. Low blood sugar profoundly affects nervous system function, including cerebral function (the part of the brain involved in reasoning, emotion, thought, memory, language, and consciousness), which over time can lead to pathological changes to the central nervous system and a variety of mental illnesses. Children experiencing stressful situations are more vulnerable to RH because stress negatively impacts blood sugar regulation. RH can be mistaken for a host of mental health conditions like anxiety, bipolar disorder, ADHD, and depression.[31]

If your child experiences the symptoms of RH between meals, tests should be run to determine how well she regulates her blood sugar. RH is diagnosed by measuring the amount of glucose in a person's blood while they are displaying symptoms and by observing if the symptoms and low blood sugar levels resolve after eating. Glucose results below 70 mg/dL may prompt the health-care professional to order a mixed meal tolerance test. During this test, your child will drink a high-calorie beverage that contains protein, carbohydrates, and fat. Blood sugar, insulin, and proinsulin levels are evaluated before the test and every thirty minutes after drinking the beverage for five hours. Lower than normal levels likely indicate RH.

Dietary adjustments are the key to managing reactive hypoglycemia. A well-balanced diet that includes more protein (protein helps stabilize blood sugar), high-fiber foods, and an abundance of fresh fruits and vegetables are the cornerstone. Sugary and highly processed foods should be limited, especially consuming these on an empty stomach. Another approach is to eat several small meals and snacks throughout the day—not allowing more than three hours to lapse between eating—without increasing your total caloric intake above your daily caloric needs.

FAMILY HISTORY OF MENTAL ILLNESS & FAMILY LIFE

Parental mental health is also a contributing factor to DMDD. Indeed, home life in general can impact the risk of DMDD. Children exposed to a chaotic home life, inconsistent attention from caregivers, or abuse are more likely to have DMDD. Maternal depression during pregnancy or during the first few months following birth increases a child's odds of developing a mood disorder, including DMDD.[32] This continues as the child grows, with children whose mothers are distressed experiencing nearly a fivefold increased risk of childhood mental health problems.[33] This is not a strictly maternal phenomenon. Research shows that poor mental health among parents—mothers and fathers—or primary caregivers is linked with poor mental and physical health in the children they care for.[34] Furthermore, parental mental health problems can have a major impact on a child's risk of behavioral, social, emotional, and educational problems.[35] A child's mental health is directly connected to and supported by their parents. Through their parents, children learn healthy social skills and how to cope with life's problems. If parents have modeled inappropriate responses to life situations, these behavioral patterns can be learned. Parents should seek counseling and support groups to manage their mental health not only for their own benefit but for that of their children.

HEAVY METALS

Heavy metals are found all around us—in our soil, water, fruits and vegetables, pipes at home, foods (including baby foods), and medications. Avoiding exposure to heavy metals simply isn't possible, but we can limit exposure and their detrimental effects. The effects of heavy metals are more severe among children compared to adults. Unfortunately, they are not easily removed from the body through its normal elimination channels, suggesting that most people could benefit from a heavy metal detox on a regular basis.

Levels of toxic heavy metals in the brain play an underrecognized role in mental illnesses and behavioral problems. Neurological damage caused by exposure to toxic metals—lead, aluminum, mercury, copper, and arsenic—may also promote aggressive, antisocial, and violent behaviors.

Examination of children's behavior and their heavy metal burden found that children with high blood-lead levels were more commonly reported to have behavioral problems like aggression, hyperactivity, and be antisocial.[36] The higher the blood-lead levels, the worse the behavior. A significant source of aluminum exposure in children is vaccinations. Many vaccines use aluminum adjuvants, and the route aluminum enters the body influences its toxic potential. Ingested aluminum is poorly soluble allowing for its effective excretion by the kidneys and through sweating. However, nearly all intramuscularly injected aluminum (like vaccine adjuvants) is absorbed into systemic circulation, and some of it travels to distant locations, such as the brain. Aluminum toxicity can disrupt nervous system function and lead to behavioral and mental health issues.[37]

Mercury interferes with brain development during childhood and adolescence, slowing electrical signals vital for communication, which gets progressively worse with age.[38] Even low levels of prenatal and childhood exposure to mercury causes both psychological and behavioral problems in children.[39,40]

Modern diets provide more copper than the recommended daily allowances (RDA), which over time can damage the liver, kidneys, heart, and brain. Common dietary sources of copper include nuts, seeds, pork, soy, raisins, avocado, dried beans, instant breakfast beverages, potatoes, dark chocolate, peanut butter, liver, oysters, and spirulina. Furthermore, humans consume high levels of copper because of copper-containing pipes and fixtures in some water distribution systems that allow copper to leach into the water. High copper levels and copper toxicity is associated with fibromyalgia, chronic fatigue, Wilson's disease, headaches, and more. Copper competes with zinc for absorption sites in the small intestine, which could lead to zinc insufficiency or deficiency. Zinc is an essential mineral involved in cellular metabolism, over 300 enzymatic reactions, immune function, wound healing, cell signaling and division, and protein and DNA synthesis. It turns out that zinc also plays a role in mood, stress responses, and cognitive function. Excess copper in the diet and through water sources can lead to inadequate levels of zinc, increasing the occurrence of depression, ADHD, aggression, anger, and violence.[41,42] Copper toxicity will likely require chelation therapy or even stomach pumping and hemodialysis. This makes it prudent to be proactive in eliminating copper from the body. It may be worth trying a low copper diet and zinc supplementation (zinc amino acid chelate)—as determined by a blood test with dosages based on level of deficiency—to see if your child's symptoms improve.

Copper toxicity can also cause neurological problems, including depression, anxiety, and overall social well-being because it decreases the availability of nutrients needed for serotonin production.[43] It is somewhat of a two-edged sword because you need enough copper to release endorphins and neurochemicals—serotonin, adrenaline, dopamine, tryptamine, noradrenaline, melatonin—that encourage feelings of love and euphoria, but too much is detrimental to emotional health. Interestingly, swimmers may be at a greater risk of heavy metal toxicity because chlorine interferes with the ability of the body to excrete copper, increasing the risk of copper toxicity.

The toxic effects of arsenic are well known, and this includes damage to nervous system function. Research shows that people with higher levels of arsenic in their blood are more likely to experience mental illness like depression and behavioral disorders.[44,45,46] Heavy metal toxicity is an oft-overlooked component of the problem that leads to DMDD. In fact, heavy metal toxicity may be a leading factor in the meteoric rise in behavioral disorders among children.

To rule out heavy metals as a contributing factor to your child's DMDD, it may be worthwhile to perform testing. Three primary tests are used to assess heavy metal body burden: hair, urine, and blood testing. While each of the tests is faulty when used alone, combining techniques can provide a more accurate picture of heavy metal body burden.

Hair testing. Although popular and less invasive, assessing heavy metal load via the hair is problematic. The presence of heavy metals in the hair may reflect efficient elimination rather than a toxic buildup in the body.

Urine testing. Urine heavy metal testing shares the same shortcoming as hair testing because heavy metal presence in the urine may represent efficient elimination of heavy metals or a body burden. In addition, some urine tests use a chelating agent (like DMSA) to provoke heavy metal release and the reference ranges for this type of test are not well-developed or validated.

Blood testing. Blood testing may be the least effective test because heavy metals typically circulate in the blood for only a short time before making a home in tissues.

Evaluate your child's current detoxification and elimination efficiency prior to beginning any heavy metal detox. This would include evaluating how frequently they have a bowel movement (should be daily) and if they sweat appropriately. Infrequent bowel movements and lack of sweating can be signs of clogged or poorly functioning elimination channels, which would need to be addressed first.

Simple and safe heavy metal detoxification tips:

1) Start with the bottom of the digestive tract by cleansing your child's colon. Psyllium husks are a good fiber option to get the bowels moving. Give your child 1.5 to 15 grams (6 to 11 years) or 2.5 to 30 grams (12 to 17 years) per day in divided doses in at least eight ounces of

water per dose. Children two years and older can use senna for up to one week as follows—4.3 mg sennosides daily (maximum 8.6 mg/day) age 2 to 5 years; 8.6 mg sennosides daily (maximum 17.2 mg/day) age 6 to 11 years; and 17.2 mg sennosides daily (maximum 34.4 mg/day) age 12 to 17 years. Do not use senna if your child has abdominal pain, intestinal obstruction, diarrhea, or acute intestinal inflammation.

2) Cleanse your child's liver with herbs like dandelion root, milk thistle, and turmeric. Seek healthcare professional guidance for dosage based on your child's current health, size, and weight.

3) Incorporate cilantro (*Coriandrum sativum* leaf) and chlorella (*Chlorella vulgaris*) as dietary supplements. Known as Nature's chelators (agents that bind to a heavy metal and then shuttle them to the excretory channels), cilantro and chlorella have been used traditionally to aid detoxification of heavy metals and other toxins. Add 0.5 mL (children 6 to 11 years) to 1 mL (children 12 and older) of alcohol-free cilantro or chlorella tincture to juice or water and consume daily. You may want to start by giving the tincture every other day and work up to daily use.

4) Encourage your child to drink plenty of water. Aim for half her body weight in ounces each day. For example, a child weighing fifty pounds should drink twenty-five ounces of clean, filtered water each day. Sufficient water is necessary to carry out wastes and toxins, especially during while cleansing.

5) Strengthen and support your child's gut with probiotics, glutamine, and quercetin.

6) Give your child Epsom salts baths with essential oils to encourage elimination through the skin. Add one to two drops each—one drop for children 2 to 8 and two drops for children 9 and older—of rosemary, cypress, and

juniper berry to half to one-cup of Epsom salts and add to warm bath water. Allow your child to soak in the water for up to twenty minutes.

7) Consider an infrared sauna to enhance your child's detoxification processes. An infrared sauna delivers light that penetrates the body to increase blood flow and oxygen levels, which can aid detoxification and reduce body aches. Aim for twenty minutes, three times a week.

Be aware that heavy metal detoxification can initially produce some adverse effects as your child reduces his heavy metal load. This includes mild flu-like symptoms, nausea, diarrhea or constipation, skin rash, lethargy, fatigue, mental fog, sleep trouble, and headaches. While these are uncomfortable, they are generally a good sign that your child's elimination channels are doing their jobs efficiently. These effects should diminish after a few days, and in the end your child will feel much better due to a reduction in his toxic burden.

ALTERED BRAIN STRUCTURE & FUNCTION

An outsider or a person who doesn't understand may view your child as simply disobedient or misbehaving, but the reality is that distorted brain structure, function, and processing is at least partly responsible. Alterations in brain structure and function have been observed in children with DMDD. One study found that children who exhibited high levels of irritability displayed a higher-than-normal level of activity in the frontal-striatal region of the brain when they were exposed to a frustrating situation.[47] This part of the brain receives inputs from dopaminergic, serotonergic, noradrenergic, and cholinergic cell groups that regulate information processing. It is involved in attention, impulse control, mood, behavior, and reward processing. Unfortunately, this aberrant neurological activity was not corrected by drugs used to treat ADHD, suggesting they may not be helpful to control chronic irritability. Another study identified brain structural changes in cortical thickness, gray matter volume, and local gyrification index (a measure of alterations in cerebral cortex development) in youths with severe irritability when compared to their healthy peers.[48] The cerebral cortex is the outer layer of the brain tissue of the cerebrum of the brain. In humans, it is typically 2.3 to 2.8 mm thick, and decreased cortical thickness in the right hemisphere disturbs arousal, attention, memory, and social stimuli, which can disrupt mood. Neuroimaging studies also show reduced gray matter volume makes individuals more susceptible to mental illness and behavioral disorder.[49,50,51] Altered local gyrification index is associated with autism, ADHD, and depression.[52,53,54] These structural deficits in the right superior frontal gyrus—an area of the brain involved in aggression and impulse control—could impede impulse control and increase irritability. Thus far, abnormal neural pattern activation and reduced activity in the reward center of the brain have been identified as brain factors that may impact the occurrence of DMDD. Essentially, children with DMDD need to work harder to control themselves when frustrated.

IMPAIRMENTS IN INSTRUMENT LEARNING & REVERSAL LEARNING

Reduced ability to adapt to and learn from life experiences is also a factor in children with DMDD. Considered a core deficit in youth with persistent aggression or irritability, impairments in instrument learning—the ability to learn from rewards and consequences—as well as shortfalls in reversal learning—the ability to adapt to changing stimuli—have been observed.[55] Thomas Jefferson was right when he defined insanity as "doing the same thing over and over and expecting different results." The honest expectation of children with DMDD is that they will have different outcomes than previously despite doing the exact same thing again. Combine this with a lack of learning from stimuli typically experienced in life, and it's easy to understand why children with DMDD must be taught or told the same thing repeatedly. An enhanced sensitivity to loss may also drive over-the-top emotional responses.[56] Based on this, Sally may feel like the world is falling apart if she has her screen time reduced after refusing to clean her room. Or she may be elated when Dad takes her out for ice cream when she performs well on her math test. In other words, a child with DMDD will overreact in her response to both rewards and consequences. She may also fixate on them. For example, continuing to ask over and over again about when she will receive the promised reward or bringing up a past punishment repeatedly.

HOSTILE INTERPRETATION BIAS

Another attribute shared among youth with DMDD that has a causal effect is errors in brain processing that lead to the inability to accurately identify facial cues, statements, and expressions.[57] Children with DMDD can easily misinterpret social situations or things said to them because of the inability to filter and process the words, actions, and emotions of others. Youth with DMDD may mistake a neutral comment or inoffensive teasing as disapproval. Constructive criticism, or even pointing out a mistake in a gentle manner, can quickly make your child defensive or argumentative. In a way, your child is wired to match what he just encountered with an expected response stored in his brain without the key context of understanding what the other person in the situation is thinking or feeling. Unable to interpret other people's behavior, he doesn't know what to say or how to behave in the mysterious situation. Successfully navigating through the social constraints requires empathy and understanding for others, not just logic.

Studies have identified abnormalities in the activation of the left or right amygdala (areas of the brain key to regulating emotions) while interpreting faces and emotions in youth with DMDD, but other research has not found this same anomaly.[58,59,60,61] Hostile interpretation bias (HIB), the tendency to interpret ambiguous social cues as threatening, inclines children with DMDD to bouts of anger and aggression in situations that are not truly a threat. If youth with DMDD do wrongly perceive neutral faces and emotions as hostile to them, it is no wonder that they treat normal situations as a threat and respond accordingly.

Imagine being in complete darkness and hearing a noise moving toward you. Without visual cues, you cannot determine if what is approaching you is a friend or foe. The logical thing to do, and what our fight-or-flight response is hardwired to do, is treat the oncoming noise as a threat until proven otherwise. This describes how children with DMDD are behaving. Without the ability to definitively prove whether a person is a friend or foe, or a situation is safe or dangerous, they default to foe and dangerous in many interactions.

DIFFICULTY PROCESSING SENSORY INFORMATION

In addition to perceptual biases toward threatening faces, DMDD youths have difficulty processing other sensations like touch, smell, taste, sound, body movement, or body position. Sensory processing is a neurological process that relies on information provided by sensory receptors regarding external and internal sensations, and then organizes and interprets these sensations to effectively coordinate muscular and emotional responses. Deciding how and with what intensity to respond to these sensations is called modulation. Healthy modulation requires maintaining a balance between habituation (decreased responses to more familiar stimuli and sensations) and sensitization (an increased or sustained reaction to a stimuli perceived as significant or threatening). Difficulty discriminating information received from sensations can lead to abnormal patterns of sensory processing and subsequently emotional and behavioral dysregulation.

In Winnie Dunn's sensory processing model, four sensory processing patterns are recognized at the intersection of threshold and the ability to control the behavioral response: (1) low registration (high threshold/passive self-regulation; it takes more intense, frequent, and longer duration sensory input and information to feel regulated when compared to neurotypical children); (2) sensory seeking (high thresholds/active self-regulation; require a near insatiable amount of sensory input to feel regulated); (3) sensory sensitivity (low thresholds/passive self-regulation; feels overwhelmed by sensory information but do not actively seek to avoid the stimulation); and (4) sensory avoiding (low thresholds/active self-regulation; feels overwhelmed by sensory information and actively avoids stimulation). All patterns of sensory processing patterns are observed in DMDD youths: sensory avoiding (40%), low registration (27%), sensory sensitivity (20%), and sensory seeking (10%).[62] It doesn't have to be only one pattern in your child. He may display parts of two or more patterns depending on the situation—familiar setting versus unfamiliar environment. Since the majority of DMDD youths are sensory avoiding, they may be described as overly sensitive because they experience sensory input more intensely than neurotypicals and strive to avoid it as they feel overwhelmed. DMDD youths, therefore, have significantly greater deficits in processing sensory information making them more prone to misread situations and other people.

For example, if your son's modulation is sensitized and under persistent sensory overload, he may perceive his environment as a constant state of danger—a figurative war zone that requires constant vigilance and escapes from peril. In other words, he has met his threshold (the amount of stimuli required to stimulate a nervous system reaction) and lost the ability to self-regulate his behavioral response to the stimuli. The concept of "making mountains out of mole hills" applies in this situation, but in your son's mind, it is a literal mountain and not a mole hill.

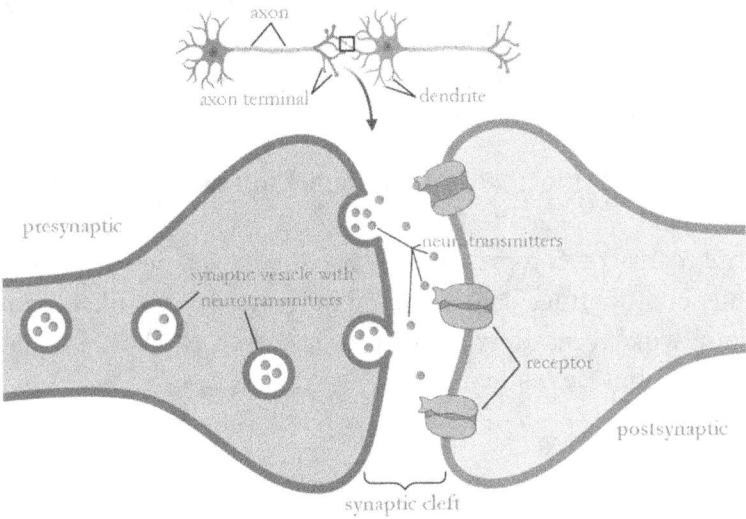

Virtually all children diagnosed with DMDD have a family history of mental illness, such as depression or anxiety, or substance abuse disorders in their family background. Currently unidentified genetic variants may make DMDD moderately heritable.[63,64] One proposed gene that may contribute to DMDD is the serotonin transporter SLC6A4 gene, which is responsible for serotonin reuptake. Brain cells communicate through signals sent to one another via neurotransmitters, like serotonin. Neurotransmitters are released from the axon and must travel across a small gap—called a synapse—to dock with receptors on other neurons to transmit information. Before neurons can send another signal, they must reabsorb (travel back across the synapse where they can be taken back into the axon) and recycle the neurotransmitters they released. This process is called reuptake. Serotonin's effect on mood is why it is a frequent target of agents designed to treat or manage mood disorders. Another gene that may have a connection to DMDD is FKBP5. This gene works with glucocorticoid receptors to help regulate the stress response. Variants in FKBP5 have been associated with multiple mood disorders, including PTSD, bipolar disorder, aggression, and suicide.[65] However, remember that genetics predispose but do not predestine a child to a DMDD outcome. Instead, lifestyle and environmental experiences act as triggers and play a substantial role in the development of DMDD in those who are predisposed by genetics.

There are several factors that contribute to the development of DMDD and its characteristic symptoms. Based on this, it is important that a comprehensive plan be developed to attack various contributing factors. Doing so increases the likelihood that you will successfully manage your child's DMDD and that he will manifest fewer symptoms.

2

TREATMENT AND MEDICATIONS

Few DMDD-specific treatment options exist in Western medicine because it is a relatively newly classified mood disorder and clinical research is lacking. Because of this, treatments are primarily based on clinical research focused on other disorders like ADHD, depression, and anxiety. The first-line treatment is typically psychotherapy (talk therapy; cognitive behavioral therapy), and medications if needed. However, sometimes psychotherapy and medication are started at the same time.

COGNITIVE BEHAVIORAL THERAPY

A principal psychotherapy used for DMDD is cognitive behavioral therapy (CBT), which helps youth learn to better cope with thoughts and feelings that contribute to their emotional outbursts. CBT may include exposure to situations that frustrate the child so they can learn to respond to those situations in a healthier way without resorting to an outburst of anger. Coping skills to control anger and ways to identify and more accurately distinguish distorted perceptions are also taught. CBT should include identification of anger triggers and strategies to prevent outbursts, social problem-solving skills, conflict resolution with parents and siblings, effective communication tactics, and role-playing of real-life social situations. Case reports do suggest that CBT can be an effective treatment for DMDD, but more research is necessary to confirm.[66,67,68] Virtually anyone who has attended therapy can tell you that finding the right therapist takes trial and error. He or she should be chosen based on the therapy type and experience with DMDD, but trying out several therapists is a normal part of the process for many youth until the *right* one is found that your child clicks with.

DIALECTIC BEHAVIOR THERAPY

Dialectical behavior therapy for children (DBT-C) was developed as a therapy to address the treatment needs of children with severe emotional dysregulation and the subsequent behavioral outbursts. For DMDD, DBT-C seeks to help children find better ways to deal with their intense emotions, learn adaptive coping skills, grasp effective problem-solving, and how parents can create a validating and safe environment that reduces their child's destabilization.

FAMILY & PARENT THERAPY

Family and parent therapy (also called parent training) is also important. Parents should seek a therapist who can help them discover effective ways to anticipate events or situations that may trigger an outburst, seek to avert it, find better ways to respond to irritable behaviors, and consider contingencies to adapt to their youth's behavior. Parent therapy should also share the importance of consistent parenting and appropriate rewards and consequences for positive and negative behaviors in a child with DMDD. One small study found that cognitive therapy for the child and parent therapy, along with stimulant medications, significantly improves depression, mood, and global functioning (the ability to meet the social and psychological demands of living), while reducing externalizing behaviors in children with DMDD and ADHD.[69] With parent therapy, parents are adequately equipped to proactively manage their child's mood and behavior. Ask your child's therapist for referrals to parent therapy.

COMPUTER-BASED TRAINING

A newer approach is computer-based training (CoBT) and focuses on a tendency of youth with DMDD to misinterpret situations, particularly facial expressions. Youth with DMDD are more likely than their peers to have information-processing deficits causing them to misperceive uncertain emotional expressions or experiences as negative.[70] Believing that an ambivalent emotional expression is angry, they treat the person as a threat and respond aggressively. For example, if Joe has DMDD, he is more likely to interpret a neutral facial expression as angry and become irritable himself. A small study reported that CoBT shifts the assessment of ambiguous faces from negative to happy in youth with DMDD.[71] Parents also reported less irritability from their children after completion of the training. Youth with DMDD are also more likely to perceive a nonhostile corrective statement, such as "Tommy, you forgot to put your dishes in the dishwasher," as a statement on their abilities and believe their parent thinks they are "stupid" or incapable of doing the dishes correctly. CoBT seeks to help children with DMDD accurately identify emotions and situations, and process facial expressions more appropriately, which can reduce defensive mechanisms that lead to outbursts.

Currently, there are no FDA-approved medications specifically for treating DMDD, but health-care providers repurpose and prescribe existing medications such as stimulants, antidepressants, and atypical antipsychotics. In many ways, pharmaceutical treatment of DMDD is like throwing spaghetti on a wall to see what sticks. Additionally, they are not really treating the root cause of the illness (because this is currently unknown) and simply masking symptoms. These drugs tend to produce mixed results in research and clinical practice because they involve so much experimentation to see what will and will not work. That being said, sometimes medication can dramatically change your child's behavior and subsequently improve family dynamics. All medications should be used based on risks versus benefits. If the benefits outweigh the risks, including parental sanity, they can be an option for your child with DMDD. However, if you are concerned about the side effects of the medications used, some of which are serious and long-lasting, effective natural solutions will be described in the next chapter.

STIMULANTS

Given that virtually all youth with DMDD also have ADHD, it is not surprising that stimulants like methylphenidate (Ritalin, Concerta) are commonly prescribed. One theory is that ADHD is caused by imbalance of the neurotransmitters dopamine and norepinephrine in the brain. Stimulants work by increasing dopamine levels in the brain, which subsequently improves attention, alertness, and energy, and reduces hyperactivity and impulsivity. However, their efficacy for DMDD is questionable and mixed at best. While stimulant medications were associated with a significant reduction in externalizing symptoms— problems with self-control of emotions and behaviors—in children with both ADHD and DMDD, only small improvements in mood were observed, and most children still experienced significant impairment, suggesting additional treatment is necessary to improve overall functioning and quality of life.[72] Additionally, some research shows that nearly one-fifth of children with DMDD who take stimulant medications experience worsened symptoms.[73] This means your child has roughly a 20 percent chance of becoming worse on the stimulant drug rather than improving. It is possible that improvements in DMDD observed in children taking stimulants are caused by improvements in co-occurring ADHD symptoms, in turn, reducing irritability.

Other stimulant medications that may be prescribed include dexmethylphenidate (Focalin), lisdexamfetamine (Vyvanse), and dextroamphetamine (Dexedrine Spansule, ProCentra).

Children taking stimulant medications should be monitored for changes in heart rate or blood pressure regularly. Stimulant medications can be habit-forming, and they should not be stopped without talking to a physician. Serious side effects that require emergency medical treatment include fast, pounding, or irregular heartbeat, chest pain, shortness of breath, seizure, slow or difficult speech, fainting, limb weakness, changes in or blurred vision, hallucinations, and difficulty breathing or swallowing. Other side effects include nervousness, irritability, mood changes, dizziness, nausea or vomiting, sleep disturbance, weight loss or loss of appetite, stomach pain, heartburn, diarrhea, headache, dry mouth, muscle tightness or pain, back pain, drowsiness, restlessness, uncontrollable movement, hives, rash, fever, and heavy sweating.

NON-STIMULANTS

Guanfacine (Intuniv, Tenex) is a long-acting nonstimulant medication used for ADHD that had previously been used to treat high blood pressure. It is approved as both a stand-alone and adjunctive (with a stimulant medication) treatment for ADHD and is used off-label for DMDD. Guanfacine's mechanism of action is not fully understood, but preclinical research suggests it may be related to stimulating neurons in the midbrain and prefrontal cortex. A small clinical study compared telepsychiatry with guanfacine in six-to-nine-year-old children with DMDD.[74] The medication group showed improvements in the frequency but not intensity of rage episodes, but experienced excessive sleepiness and stomach pain. Telepsychiatry was also effective, suggesting psychotherapy may be a preferred first-line treatment for DMDD.

Intuniv is only approved for children six years old and older. Call the prescribing physician if your child experiences serious side effects such as anxiety, nervousness, irregular or slow heartbeat, pain or tightness in the chest, hallucinations, lightheadedness, difficulty breathing, increased urinary frequency, or severe drowsiness. Some parents report their children have nightmares or display increased violent tendencies on guanfacine. Commonly reported adverse reactions include dizziness, drowsiness, blurred vision, confusion, lightheadedness upon standing, low blood pressure, slow heartbeat, irritability, tiredness, sleep disturbance, stomach pain, nausea, constipation, sweating, and dry mouth.

ANTIDEPRESSANTS

Selective norepinephrine reuptake inhibitors (SNRIs) are prescribed to treat irritability and depression. A prototype SNRI, venlafaxine (Effexor) failed to reduce irritability compared to placebo in a small study of thirteen people with autism and irritability symptoms.[75] However, a decrease in behavioral problems and aggression was noted in the venlafaxine group. Atomoxetine (Strattera) is another SNRI approved to treat ADHD that may be prescribed for DMDD when children fail to respond to or are intolerant to stimulants. Four randomized clinical trials have been conducted with atomoxetine in children with aggressive behavior diagnosed with ADHD and comorbid ODD, depression, or anxiety. Overall, atomoxetine exerted a small effect, causing researchers to state it may not be an optimal medication for pediatric aggression given such a small effect over a long period.[76]

A selective serotonin reuptake inhibitor (SSRI) antidepressant, fluoxetine (Prozac, Sarafem) may be prescribed for DMDD. A preliminary trial began in 2013 to study the effects of lisdexamfetamine combined with fluoxetine.[77] Subjects first received lisdexamfetamine titrated until an optimal dose was achieved. Then participants were randomized to add fluoxetine or placebo for eight weeks. However, no conclusions were found regarding the efficacy of the trial despite its completion in 2016. Of the published findings on fluoxetine, one showed no effect on aggressive behaviors, while other research suggests that combining fluoxetine with CBT is superior to either treatment option alone.[78] The lack of significant clinical efficacy for SNRI and SSRI antidepressants in children with DMDD seems to indicate they are not great options to treat DMDD.

SNRIs and SSRIs carry the sternest FDA "black box" warning because of their association with suicidal thoughts and behaviors among young people. Additionally, observational research has linked antidepressants to a moderately increased risk of homicidal ideation and violence toward others.[79,80] Common adverse effects of these drugs include constipation, diarrhea, loss of appetite, dizziness, nausea, vomiting, dry mouth, drowsiness, headache, insomnia, stomach upset, agitation, anxiousness, shakiness, and hot flashes. SNRIs or SSRIs may cause discontinuation syndrome—a group of symptoms (insomnia, nightmares, vivid dreams, dizziness, vertigo, loss of muscle coordination, numbness or tingling in areas of the body, lethargy, headache tremor, sweating, irritability, anxiety, agitation, and depression) that occur after abrupt discontinuation of certain drugs—when stopped suddenly, so they should be withdrawn slowly and under a health-care professionals guidance.

Bupropion (Wellbutrin, Zyban) is an atypical antidepressant most commonly used as an add-on medication when people have an incomplete response to other antidepressants. Its mechanism of action is not fully understood, although it is believed to be related to weak inhibition of the reuptake of dopamine and norepinephrine. Three separate studies, totaling a hundred youth, measuring the effects of bupropion for aggressive behavior concluded that it had no or a modest effect.[81] The tricyclic antidepressant desipramine (Norpramin) had the greatest effect on aggressive behavior in children and adolescents with ADHD according to a meta-analysis.[82] This drug works by selectively blocking the reuptake of norepinephrine (noradrenaline) and to a lesser extent serotonin reuptake. Inhibition of the reuptake of these neurotransmitters leads to increased signaling by the neurotransmitter. Research included sixty-two youths with ADHD, forty-three of whom previously responded poorly to stimulant medications.[83] At the conclusion of the six-week study, 68 percent of youth receiving desipramine were very much or much improved and the medication was well tolerated. However, the shortcoming of reuptake inhibiting drugs is that they expose the neurotransmitters to enzymes designed to degrade them. Over time, reuptake inhibitors can cause further depletion of neurotransmitters and the drug's effects diminish, causing the person to feel worse.

Although an atypical antidepressant, like most antidepressants, bupropion has a "black box" warning because of an increased risk of suicidal ideation or behavior in children and youth. Common adverse effects include anxiety, restlessness, shaking, difficulty sleeping, irregular heartbeat, dry mouth, and hyperventilation. Less commonly people taking bupropion may experience ringing in the ears, severe headache, hives, skin rash, or itching. Rare side effects include anger, violent behavior, chest pain, inability to sit still, fast or pounding heartbeat, or overexcitement.

ANTIPSYCHOTICS

Risperidone (Risperdal) is an atypical antipsychotic used to treat bipolar disorder and schizophrenia that is also used for DMDD. Like many psychiatric drugs used, its mechanism is not completely understood but it may be related to interactions with dopamine and serotonin receptors. A small open-label clinical trial (twenty-one children with severe mood dysregulation) reported that taking risperidone reduced atypical behaviors, irritability, ADHD symptoms, depression, and improved global functioning.[84] A larger study evaluated the effects of risperidone among children with severe physical aggression, ADHD, and oppositional defiance disorder who were already taking a stimulant drug and whose parents received parent training.[85] The drug cocktail and parent training produced greater behavioral, social, and total clinical outcomes than standard treatment alone. Elevated prolactin—suggesting it may be disrupting endocrine system function—and upset stomach were commonly reported in the combination treatment group. Of concern with risperidone and any antipsychotic drug, is their potential to cause an imbalance in brain chemistry.

Aripiprazole (Abilify) is an atypical antipsychotic medication primarily used to treat bipolar disorder and schizophrenia. It is also used to treat irritability, aggression, temper tantrums, and mood swings in children with autism. Based on its effectiveness for the mentioned symptoms, clinicians have used the drug to treat DMDD. It too interacts with dopamine and serotonin receptors in the brain seeking to restore neurochemical balance. It has been used with stimulant drugs in small clinical trials. A

2009 small (sixteen children) study assessed the use of aripiprazole with methylphenidate among children with what was then called pediatric bipolar disorder and ADHD. Depressive symptoms were reduced, but ADHD symptoms and manic episodes were not different than placebo.[86] One subject withdrew from the trial because of significant mood disturbances caused by the combined treatment. An open-label pilot study (twenty-four children with DMDD and ADHD) evaluated the effectiveness of taking aripiprazole with methylphenidate.[87] The combination treatment improved irritability, externalizing symptoms, depression, anxiety, attention, and social problems. Another study found that aripiprazole was no better than placebo in reducing irritability in children with autism.[88] Even though some effect was observed in these studies, the long-term safety of taking this drug cocktail that transforms brain chemistry is not proven.

A meta-analysis looked at the efficacy and side effect risks of risperidone and aripiprazole for behavioral disturbances in children with autism or intellectual disabilities and found that they were similar in efficacy but associated with frequent side effects.[89] The most common side effects were weight gain, extrapyramidal syndrome (drug-induced movement disorders such as involuntary or uncontrollable movements, tremors, or muscle contractions), and excessiveness tiredness/sleepiness.

An antipsychotic drug formerly widely used to treat schizophrenia and psychosis, thioridazine (Mellaril, Melleril), was studied in children with adolescent conduct disorder (ACD) in the early 1990s.[90] The branded drug was withdrawn from the market worldwide in 2005 due to its association with severe cardiac arrhythmias, but generic versions are still available and used in the United States. The study found that thioridazine had only minor behavioral effects and was inferior to methylphenidate based on teacher ratings of problem behavior and absolute efficacy. Thioridazine also blocks dopamine receptors, which is intended to treat the positive symptoms of schizophrenia, such as delusions and hallucinations. Based on its limited efficacy and significant safety risks, thioridazine appears to have no place in the treatment of DMDD.

Another atypical antipsychotic medication, quetiapine (Seroquel) has been investigated in youth with ACD. ACD is a mental health condition where children and teens engage in a consistent pattern of aggressive behaviors and actions that harm the well-being of others and consistently violate societal norms and rules. This pilot study found that quetiapine worked better than placebo for improving symptoms and behaviors associated with ACD when assessed by the clinician.[91] Yet, the parents did not notice significant difference when surveyed. Additionally, one of five youths receiving quetiapine had to withdraw from the trial because he developed akathisia—a movement disorder characterized by a persistent feeling of inner restlessness, mental distress, and the inability to remain still. Quetiapine interacts with many receptors in the brain and, like other antipsychotics, attempts to block dopamine to reduce symptoms.

Haloperidol (Haldol) is a first-generation antipsychotic that works by rebalancing dopamine levels in the brain, which improves mood, thinking, and behavior. Two studies found that haloperidol was effective in alleviating behavioral symptoms in youth with autism.[92,93] No side effects were noted during the treatment.

The type and occurrence of side effects caused by antipsychotics depends on the medication, dosage, and frequency of taking it. Most common are weight gain, digestive issues, drowsiness, blurry vision, dizziness, restlessness, mental fog, loss of motivation, social withdrawal, altered metabolism, metabolic syndrome, type 2 diabetes, and uncontrollable movements.

Valproate sodium (Valproate, Depakote) is an anticonvulsant drug approved to control seizures, prevent migraines, and treat bipolar disorder by altering certain chemicals in the brain. Three studies evaluated its effectiveness in managing the cardinal symptoms of DMDD, including aggression, explosive temper, and disrupted mood. The largest of the three studies found that it had no statistically significant effect when compared to placebo.[94] Conversely, the two smaller studies showed a reduction in anger, hostility, and irritability.[95,96] Two additional anticonvulsants approved for bipolar disorder and neurotic pain treatment respectively, lamotrigine (Lamictal) and carbamazepine (Tegretol) did not help reduce the targeted symptoms of DMDD in clinical research.[97,98] The totality of the available research suggests that anticonvulsants do not improve DMDD.

Valproate is associated with the following common side effects: nausea, vomiting, headache, hair loss, weight gain, diarrhea, abdominal pain, drowsiness, dizziness, and muscle weakness. Rare but serious side effects include liver damage, low platelets, pancreatitis, and elevated ammonia levels. Research suggests that people taking anticonvulsants have suicidal thoughts and behaviors roughly twice as often as people taking a placebo— affecting about one in five hundred individuals.[99]

Since DMDD was once confused with pediatric bipolar disorder, lithium has been tried as a treatment because of its successful treatment of bipolar disorder. Lithium is a mood stabilizer that helps decrease the intensity of manic episodes and reduces the severity of depressive episodes. However, no clinically significant improvement in DMDD symptoms was noted in several clinical studies.[100,101,102] In fact, one study found that the lithium was no more effective than placebo.[103] The current evidence does not support the use of lithium for DMDD.

Side effects of lithium include hypothyroidism, confusion, poor memory, fainting, irregular or pounding heartbeat, frequent urination, increased thirst, trouble breathing (especially during exertion), weight gain, and excessive tiredness or weakness. Rarely, vision or hearing problems, eye pain, dizziness, blue color of toes or fingers, coldness of limbs, or headache occur.

Naltrexone (Revia) is a medication used for alcohol or opioid abuse that is also used for a variety of autoimmune conditions at much lower doses than those used for drug withdrawal symptoms. It has also been used at the higher dose for DMDD. A case report of a fifteen-year-old boy with DMDD and ADHD reports the use of 50 mg/day of naltrexone after methylphenidate, guanfacine, and aripiprazole all failed to control his symptoms.[104] The boy's aggression and symptoms improved with the treatment. Due to a lack of evidence for the long-term use of naltrexone for DMDD, the drug was discontinued after three months, and the aggressive symptoms resumed. Reintroduction of naltrexone improved his symptoms again. Insufficient evidence exists to know whether naltrexone could play a role in the treatment of DMDD, but it may be worth discussing with your health-care professional if other treatments have failed to produce results.

Some of the most common adverse reactions of naltrexone include sleep disturbance, vivid dreams or nightmares, headache, dry mouth or throat, nausea, upset stomach, and increased heart rate. Less commonly, anxiety, fatigue, loss of appetite, mood swings, shortness of breath, agitation, dizziness, increased hair growth, and disorientation occur. Naltrexone can cause liver damage at higher doses, but this is less common at lower doses.

A meta-analysis of eighteen randomized controlled clinical trials found that psychotropic medications—stimulants, SNRIs, antipsychotics, mood stabilizers, beta blockers, alpha-2 agonists, and antidepressants—had a moderate to large effect on aggressive behaviors in children with methylphenidate being the most effective for aggressive behavior co-occurring with ADHD and risperidone for persistent behavioral disturbances in children with conduct disorders and a below average IQ.[105] However, the analysis noted that longer-duration studies with better methodologies are needed.

3

NATURAL SOLUTIONS

Just like the drugs used for DMDD, there isn't a clinically proven natural solution for DMDD. However, herbs and dietary supplements have been used for decades to support and restore health, and many do have meaningful clinical research showing that they work by mechanisms and pathways that could benefit children and youth with DMDD. Additionally, as pharmaceutical researchers and clinicians do, evidence from clinical research on related conditions can be leveraged to help guide the use of supplements.

BACOPA

Commonly used in Ayurvedic medicine, bacopa (*Bacopa monneri*) may help youth with DMDD by reducing anxiety, enhancing cognitive performance, and improving mood. It is considered a nootropic—a substance that enhances cognition, especially memory and learning, improves brain cell communication, and helps the brain function under disruptive conditions—and believed to help the brain process information faster because it causes branches of nerve cells (dendrites) to grow. Dendrites are small extensions of brain cells, resembling tree roots or branches, that receive signals from other brain cells. As dendrites grow, they become thicker with a healthy myelin coating that improves brain cell signaling and communication. Other nootropics include caffeine and stimulant medications like Adderall (amphetamine, dextroamphetamine). However, unlike these stimulants, bacopa is an adaptogen and makes most people feel calmer and more socially at ease. Moreover, bacopa interacts with the dopamine, GABAergic, cholinergic, and serotonin systems,[106,107,108] reducing the depletion of dopamine and serotonin caused by prolonged stress and creating balance in brain neurotransmitters—GABA, dopamine, serotonin, and acetylcholine. With all of its beneficial effects in the brain, bacopa may restore healthy function of areas of the brain that are deficient in children with DMDD, including enhancing executive function—the cognitive processes involving one's ability to organize thoughts and activities, prioritize tasks, exercise self-control, manage time efficiently, and make decisions. Trouble with executive functions can make it hard to handle emotions, focus, and follow directions.

An open-label study found that taking 225 mg of bacopa daily for six months significantly improved ADHD symptoms (restlessness, self-control, impulsivity, and learning problems) in children aged six to twelve.[109] A later larger randomized, placebo-controlled clinical trial evaluated the effects of bacopa in children with ADHD aged six to fourteen years. Boys and male youths in the study took 160–320 mg of bacopa with breakfast depending on body weight for fourteen weeks.[110] Improvements in cognitive flexibility, executive function, interpersonal problems, and sleep were noted in those taking bacopa. Given its consistent and remarkable effects on disorders affecting the brain, bacopa is a leading and promising candidate to manage DMDD.

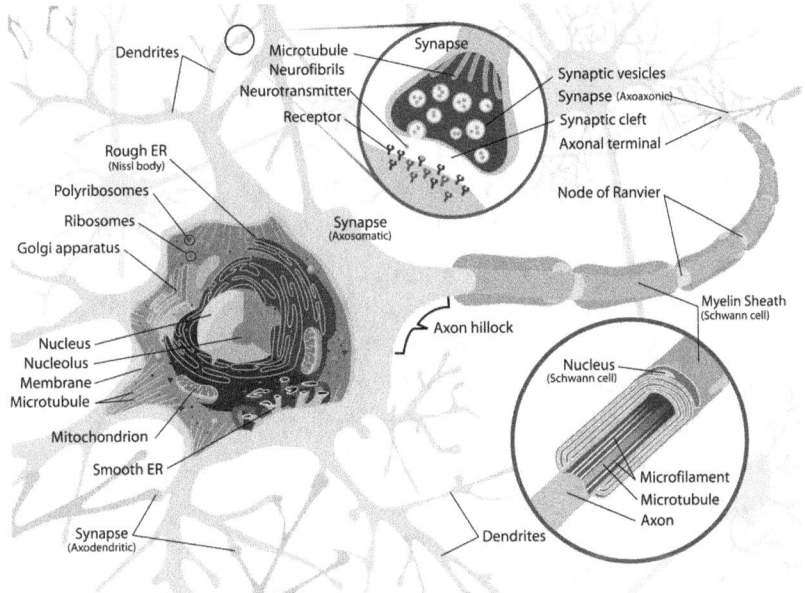

Bacopa may take four to six weeks to see results because it takes time for dendrites to grow and enhance brain cell communication.

Bacopa (standardized to ≥55% total bacosides)*

Typical dose: 300 mg, twice daily, with food; or 600 mg per day with breakfast

Contraindications: Hyperthyroidism

Ask your health-care professional or pharmacist before using: Pregnancy, lactation, bradycardia, GI obstruction, stomach ulcer, pulmonary conditions, hyperthyroidism, urogenital tract obstruction

Potential interactions: Cholinergic/anticholinergic, thyroid medications, drugs, drugs metabolized by the CYP1A2, CYP2C19, CYP2C9, and CYP3A4 enzymes

Reported adverse effects: Abdominal cramps, diarrhea, nausea, dry mouth

* Note, one clinically tested extract contained 20 percent bacosides.

PHOSPHATIDYLSERINE

Like bacopa, phosphatidylserine is a nootropic used to improve mood, memory, and learning ability, and reduce the effects of prolonged stress. It is a phospholipid created by the body and component of cell membranes, where it is concentrated on the inner surface. It is the most abundant phospholipid in the human brain and critical for neuron membrane function—maintenance of the internal cellular environment, cell-to-cell communication, and cell growth regulation. It is possible that phosphatidylserine reverses abnormalities in neuronal membranes associated with alterations in neurotransmitter functioning. Preclinical and clinical research shows that phosphatidylserine does indeed increase various neurotransmitters in the brain, including acetylcholine, norepinephrine, serotonin, and dopamine.[111,112,113] A deficit in phosphatidylserine in the basal ganglia and prefrontal cortex of children with ADHD has been noted.[114,115] These brain regions are the target of stimulant medications used for ADHD, and so researchers theorize that low phosphatidylserine levels may contribute to symptoms of ADHD. Although the body can create phosphatidylserine, enhanced benefits can be realized through supplementation.

A systemic review and meta-analysis concluded that preliminary evidence from clinical trials suggests that phosphatidylserine may be effective in reducing symptoms of ADHD, although the quality of the evidence is low and further research is necessary to make definitive conclusions.[116] It should also be noted that two of the clinical trials combined phosphatidylserine with omega-3 fatty acids, which could have influenced the results. Early evidence suggests that supplementation with phosphatidylserine may support healthy neurons and balance neurotransmitter and brain function to improve DMDD.

Phosphatidylserine
_____

Typical dose: 200–300 mg, daily, in the morning, preferably with at least 80–160 mg of EPA and 50–100 mg of DHA

Contraindications: None currently known

Ask your health-care professional or pharmacist before using: Pregnancy, lactation

Potential interactions: Anticholinergic/cholinergic meds

Reported adverse effects: Flatulence, upset stomach, headache, insomnia, nausea

N-ACETYL CYSTEINE & GLUTATHIONE

Traumatic, stressful situations, particularly during critical development periods when sensitivity to stress is heightened and neural networks are being formed (neuroplasticity), like during childhood, may over- or undersensitize nervous and endocrine system responses.[117] This neuroendocrine dysregulation can lead to altered homeostatic state fraught with disordered stress responses and a shift to survival mode. Consequently, abnormal neurobiological alterations occur, even decades after the traumatic stressor that triggered it all. One of the ways this occurs is through trauma-related oxidative stress or an unbalanced amount of free radicals to antioxidants. Ordinarily, free radical oxidants and reactive oxygen species (ROS) are efficiently neutralized by the body through a complex antioxidant defense system that involves the enzymes superoxide dismutase, catalase, and glutathione (including glutathione peroxidase and glutathione reductase). Glutathione—consisting of cysteine, glutamate, and glycine—is the most important intracellular defense mechanism against oxidative stress. A growing body of evidence suggests that oxidative stress and impaired metabolism of glutathione play a key role in the development of mental illness, including bipolar disorder, which is related to DMDD.[118] Any imbalance between antioxidant defenses and oxidants leads to oxidative damage to cells and tissues that are connected to the development of several disorders, including mental health, mood, and behavioral disorders.

One of the proposed ways to restore glutathione metabolism and overcome oxidative stress is to supplement with n-Acetyl-cysteine (NAC). NAC is an antioxidant precursor to glutathione, known to restore reduced glutathione levels.[119] Autism shares the traits of irritability and periods of excessive frustration with DMDD. Two of the hypothesized mechanisms for the symptoms of autism are oxidative stress and the subsequent accumulation of ROS.[120] A randomized, double-blind, placebo-controlled trial evaluated the effectiveness of taking NAC as an adjunct to risperidone for autism.[121] Children under 20 kg (44 lbs) took 200 mg, three times daily, whereas children 20 kg or heavier took 300 mg, three times daily. Over the course of the ten-week study, children receiving NAC demonstrated significant improvements in irritability and hyperactivity/noncompliance, which exceeded that of risperidone alone. Another study also reported a decrease in irritability in children with autism who took 600 mg of NAC, twice daily, along with risperidone.[122] Given the potential role of oxidative stress in promoting neuroendocrine dysfunction, it may be worth trying NAC supplements, particularly in younger children, to possibly prevent disrupting these critical systems or mitigate existing disruption.

n-Acetyl Cysteine
_____

Typical dose: 600 mg, twice daily; or 200–300 mg, three times daily

Contraindications: Acetyl cysteine allergy

Ask your health-care professional or pharmacist before using: Pregnancy, lactation, bleeding disorders, surgery

Potential interactions: Nitroglycerin, anticoagulant/antiplatelet drugs, activated charcoal, blood pressure meds, chloroquine; anticoagulant/antiplatelet supplements, supplements that lower blood pressure

Reported adverse effects: Diarrhea, dry mouth, heartburn, loss of appetite, nausea, vomiting; Rare: chest tightness, heart palpitations

Mood stabilizers like lithium and valproate work at least partly by increasing glutathione levels,[123] suggesting that taking glutathione directly may be of benefit in DMDD. Glutathione can be taken as an oral supplement, as long as it is the right form that is bioavailable and effective in increasing glutathione levels. Acetylglutathione (also called acetylated glutathione) is stable in the intestine and blood, where it is delivered directly to cells for deacetylation inside the cell. Ordinary glutathione (reduced glutathione, GSH) delivered to the blood by precursors like liposomes (liposomal glutathione) must be broken down into basic amino acid components by enzymes to be absorbed inside the cell. Once inside the cell, glutathione must be reconstructed back to GSH. Based on this, it appears better to take the orally active and more bioavailable form acetylglutathione to increase glutathione levels inside cells without the increasing energy expenditure to reconstruct it from its amino acid components.

S-acetylglutathione (S-Acetyl L-Glutathione)
Typical dose: 100–300 mg, daily

Contraindications: None currently known

Ask your health-care professional or pharmacist before using: None currently known

Potential interactions: None currently known

Reported adverse effects: Oral glutathione is generally well tolerated without adverse effects

Given the enormous effect gut health, specifically gut integrity and microflora, has on brain and immune function, it is reasonable to suppose that both probiotics and natural solutions designed to enhance gut integrity may have an effect on DMDD. Although separated by a great distance in the body, the brain and the gut are intricately connected and communicate regularly through small molecules, proteins, and a direct neural connection. When either the brain or the gut is disturbed, the other can be negatively influenced, leading to gastrointestinal, mood, or neurological disorders.

The gut contains its own nervous system, called the enteric nervous system (ENS), which contains millions of neurons. This system uses the vagus nerve, endocrine system hormones, and immune pathways to communicate with the brain. The ENS also regulates gut integrity, which is significantly influenced by the microbes residing in the gut. Indeed, gut microbes communicate with each other electrically through proteins called ion channels, just like neurons in the brain.[124,125] The microbes residing in the gut have such a profound effect on health, both mental and physical, that the lack of a gut microbiome can result in dramatic changes in psychophysiological functions and even alter brain physiology.[126] Changes in serotonin and brain-derived neurotrophic factor (BDNF) levels in the hippocampus, structural alterations of neurons in the amygdala, and variations in myelination in the prefrontal cortex have all been observed in the absence of a gut microbiome. These changes in brain physiology caused by an unhealthy microbiome increase the risk of anxiety, depression, and stress-related disorders as well as cognitive deficits and abnormal social behaviors. Fascinatingly, research in animals shows that simply transplanting the gut microbiota from an animal with anxiety to another can trigger anxiety in the animal receiving the transplant.[127] Moreover, preclinical research shows that serotonin production—90 percent of which is produced in the gut,[128,129] not the brain—is also heavily reliant upon gut microbes.[130] Healthy gut microbiome diversity also plays a role in dopamine production.[131,132] Drastic changes in the gut microbiome have been observed in people with many mood and cognitive disorders, illustrating the vital importance of maintaining a healthy gut microbiome.

Fortunately, emerging research suggests that certain dietary supplements can restore or strengthen your intestinal barrier, and a strong body of evidence supports supplementation with probiotics to improve microbiome diversity and quantity. Starting with microbiome diversity may be most sensible since it can also influence leaky gut. Not to mention that taking a probiotic is key to overall health as well.

The presence of bacterial toxins (endotoxins) in the bloodstream after eating is a hallmark sign of leaky gut. Called endotoxemia, this condition can increase the absorption of pathogens and toxins into the bloodstream and tissues, intensify inflammation, and contribute to mood disorders. A clinical study investigated the effects of probiotic supplementation in healthy men and women whose endotoxin concentration increased by at least fivefold after eating. The researchers found that ingestion of a spore-based probiotic supplement containing *Bacillus indicus* (HU36), *Bacillus subtilis* (HU58), *Bacillus coagulans*, *Bacillus licheniformis*, and *Bacillus clausii* for thirty days produced a 42 percent reduction in endotoxins in the bloodstream and a 24 percent reduction in triglycerides.[133] On the contrary, the placebo group that ingested a rice-flour supplement experienced increases in endotoxins (36%) and triglycerides (5%). According to this research and clinical experience, supplementing with commensal bacteria improves the strategic defenses in your gut and limits the escape of harmful substances from the gut to the bloodstream.

When healthy men ingested a supplement containing six probiotic strains—*Bifidobacterium bifidum* W23, *Bifidobacterium lactis* W51, *Enterococcus faecium* W54, *Lactobacillus acidophilus* W22, *Lactobacillus brevis* W63, and *Lactococcus lactis* W58—after intense exercise, zonulin levels decreased (suggesting improved gut integrity), protein oxidation was reduced, and inflammation declined.[134] This is further evidence of the wide-ranging benefits of improving gut microbiome diversity.

Multistrain Probiotic

Typical dose: Twenty-five billion+ CFUs initially; minimum ten billion CFUs for maintenance; as directed on the supplement label, preferably after a meal

Contraindications: Serious immunosuppression

Ask your health-care professional or pharmacist before using: Pancreatitis

Potential interactions: Should be taken at least two to four hours after antibiotics or antifungals

Reported adverse effects: Digestive upset

L-glutamine is an amino acid that plays a fundamental role in immune, digestive, muscular, intestinal health, mood, and cognition. Beyond these important functions, glutamine helps maintain healthy gut barrier function and can help correct microbiome imbalances. The cells of the intestines are replaced every few days, making it possible to heal the gut in a short period of time, perhaps only a few weeks. Glutamine enhances the production and survival of gut cells (enterocytes), speeding the process of replacing damaged cells—regrow and repair—that are allowing leakage of toxins and pathogens from the intestines to the bloodstream.[135] By supporting the health of your gut cells, glutamine helps promote tight intestinal junctions, reduce gut inflammation, and alleviate leaky gut.[136,137,138] In addition, L-glutamine may improve mood and cognition.

It is very difficult to consume enough glutamine in capsules, so it is most often taken in a free powder form that is mixed in a beverage. This may also be easier to digest and utilize.

L-Glutamine, or stabilized glutamine (L-Alanyl-L-Glutamine)
Typical dose: 5 g powder in a cold beverage, one to three times daily on an empty stomach, maximum of 15 g/day (start with 2 g per dose for the first few days and then work up to 5 g per dose)

Contraindications: None currently known

Ask your health-care professional or pharmacist before using: Pregnancy, lactation, epilepsy and other convulsive disorders, liver cirrhosis, hepatic encephalopathy

Potential interactions: Anticonvulsant drugs

Reported adverse effects: Burping, bloating, constipation, cough, diarrhea, digestive discomfort, headache, musculoskeletal pain

Chronic stress also influences intestinal permeability and mast cells—cells rich in tissue that interact with the outside world such as your skin, gastrointestinal tract, and respiratory tract—that play an important role in leaky gut.[139] Specifically, stress increases mast cell levels in intestinal mucus membranes and the number of them that are activated. Interestingly, when rats were bred to have no mast cells in the gut, they could no longer develop leaky gut.[140] Mast cells help regulate immune responses and repair tissues. Their primary role is to stimulate immune responses to toxins and pathogens. When activated, they degranulate (destabilize) and release a host of chemicals (lysosomal enzymes, histamine, heparin, serotonin, cytokines, chemokines, prostanoides, leukotrienes, and proteases) that affect innate and adaptive immune responses. These chemicals widen blood vessels, promote the creation of new blood vessels, stimulate detoxification, regulate bone growth, and influence respiratory function. While important, excess activation of mast cells or improper activation in response to harmless antigens, can promote allergies by increasing intestinal permeability and allowing molecules to escape from the digestive tract into the bloodstream.

A plant flavonoid and potent antioxidant, quercetin is found in many common foods, such as apples, grapes, berries, onions, and tea. Quercetin stabilizes mast cells, preventing their release of chemicals including histamine, and also prevents intestinal cell toxicity.[141,142,143,144] Furthermore, quercetin enhances gut barrier function because of its role in the assembly and expression of tight junction proteins and reverses imbalances in the gut microbiome.[145] This activity produces a sealing effect by connecting intestinal cells so nutrients can enter the bloodstream, but larger molecules like toxins and pathogens can't escape the digestive tract. Experimental and animal research demonstrates that quercetin reverses leaky gut, heals the digestive tract, and restores depleted glutathione.[146,147,148,149] The takeaway is that you should eat fruits and vegetables rich in quercetin and consider taking a supplement (a better choice since getting therapeutic doses from food can be very difficult unless you like eating lots of onions) to fight leaky gut and dysbiosis.

Quercetin or Quercetin LipoMicel Matrix

Typical dose: Quercetin—250 mg, two to three times daily; Quercetin LipoMicel Matrix—250 mg, once daily

Contraindications: Pregnancy

Ask your health-care professional or pharmacist before using: Lactation, bleeding disorders, kidney disorders

Potential interactions: Blood pressure meds, anticoagulant/antiplatelet meds, drugs metabolized by CYP2C8, CYP2C9, CYP2D6, and CYP3A4 enzymes, quinolone antibiotics, immunosuppressives; anticoagulant/antiplatelet supplements, supplements that affect blood pressure

Reported adverse effects: Headache, tingling of extremities

For children and youth with DMDD and co-occurring depression, and not taking medications, St. John's wort (*Hypericum perforatum*) is worthy of consideration. Extracts of St. John's wort contain napthodianthrones (including hypericin and pseudohypericin), phloroglucinols (including hyperforin), and flavonoids (like quercetin, kaempferol, and luteolin) that are responsible for its mood benefits. The most active antidepressant constituents are considered hyperforin and adhyperforin and several other related compounds.[150] This is why Perika, a St. John's wort extract standardized to hyperforin, is highly recommended. Hyperforin, adhyperforin, and their related compounds regulate serotonin, dopamine, and norepinephrine by inhibiting their reuptake.[151] Unlike the reuptake inhibitor drugs mentioned previously, the active compounds in St. John's wort are non-competitive reuptake inhibitors. This means they do not actually bind to and block reuptake transporters. Instead, they influence presynaptic sodium channels that regulate reuptake transporter activity. Visualize this process as a gate versus cement traffic barriers. Drugs act like the cement barriers by blocking travel beyond their location; whereas St. John's wort is a gate that can be opened and closed more easily, allowing some travel beyond the gate when needed. Understanding how St. John's wort works differently on neurotransmitters may explain why it is not associated with the same side effects as antidepressant drugs that competitively inhibit reuptake.

Hyperforin also influences GABA, glutamate, and beta-adrenergic activities. Adrenergic receptors are the targets of catecholamines, such as norepinephrine and epinephrine, and involved in regulating physiological responses to stress. In a complex interaction with serotonin, adrenergic receptors determine one's resilience to stress and mood dysregulation after adversity, tragedy, trauma, threat, or significant stress.

Contrarily, hypericin inhibits monoamine oxidase (MAO) type A, but it is believed that hypericin cannot reach adequate levels in the brain to produce significant effects.[152,153] Interestingly, hypericin hinders brain changes caused by stress similarly to imipramine, although to a lesser degree.[154] This suggests it may also contribute to increased resilience to stressful situations. Enhanced stress resilience may reduce the descent into mood dysregulation and outbursts seen in children with DMDD by helping them bounce back from an anxiety-provoking experience more quickly.

The primary challenge with using St. John's wort clinically is its many interactions with medications, which limit its therapeutic use. However, since it is generally effective and has fewer side effects than antidepressant medications, it may be helpful for those not taking other medications, including stimulants.

Standardized forms of St. John's wort have shown great effectiveness—as effective as SSRIs and other antidepressants—for mild to moderate depression in clinical research with fewer side effects.[155,156,157,158,159,160,161] One study evaluating St. John's wort in children under twelve years old found that it improved depression.[162] Remarkably, the number of physicians rating its effectiveness as good to excellent was 72 percent after two weeks, 97 percent after four weeks, and 100 percent after six weeks, which also suggests that it can take from four to six weeks to be fully effective. Another trial found that more than three-quarters of youths aged six to sixteen experienced improvements in moderate depressive symptoms when taking St. John's wort,[163] while a third study reported that 82 percent of youths aged twelve to seventeen showed significant clinical improvement in depression after taking St. John's wort for eight weeks.[164] The research is clear that St. John's wort is an effective, and most likely safer option, for depression.

St. John's wort has also been evaluated in children with ADHD. However, this small clinical trial did not find that it improved ADHD symptoms such as inattentiveness and hyperactivity when compared to the placebo.[165] This is not completely surprising, since the mechanisms and pathways that St. John's wort works by is more compatible with depression than ADHD.

St. John's Wort (Perika)

Typical dose: 300 mg, twice daily, at mealtime; standardized to 3 percent hyperforin (range of 1%–6%) or 0.3 percent hypericin

Contraindications: Pregnancy, lactation

Ask your health-care professional or pharmacist before using: Alzheimer's diseases, bipolar depression, schizophrenia, and before surgery

Potential interactions: Stimulants, tranquilizing drugs (Xanax), barbiturates, blood pressure, blood thinning and anticoagulant drugs, digoxin, ivabradine, anti-glioma drugs (aminolevulinic acid), protease inhibitors, antidepressants, antipsychotics, contraceptives, cyclosporine, drugs that interfere with CYP1A2, CYP2B6, CYP2C19, CYP2C9, CYP3A4, chemotherapy agents, fentanyl, allergy drugs, finasteride, antidiabetic meds, HMG-CoA reductase inhibitors, ketamine, anticonvulsants and antiseizure meds, opioids and opioid withdrawal meds, non-nucleotide reverse transcriptase inhibitors, omeprazole, p-glycoprotein substrates, photosensitizing drugs, immunosuppressive meds, theophylline, voriconazole, zolpidem; cardiac glycoside-containing herbs (digitalis), herbs and supplements that affect serotonin levels, iron supplements (may reduce absorption of iron), and red yeast rice

Reported adverse effects: Diarrhea, gastrointestinal discomfort (mild), dizziness, dry mouth, fatigue, headache, insomnia, restlessness, and sedation

Found abundantly in the cerebrum, cerebellum, brain stem, and spinal cord, gray matter is involved in movement control, emotional regulation, memory retention, decision-making, and self-control. Gray matter is the outermost layer of the brain that encases both left and right hemispheres. It is distinguished from white brain matter due to the presence of a greater number of cell bodies and fewer myelinated axons when compared to white matter. While declines in gray matter volume are observed during the aging process, those with mental illnesses tend to have a greater degree of decline. As a matter of fact, gray matter volumes can predict mental health treatment outcomes. Structural magnetic resonance imaging (MRI) scans using a machine-learning algorithm revealed distinct markers of mental illness and treatment outcomes in three hundred people with recent onset of depression or psychosis.[166] People with lower gray matter volumes experience higher levels of cognitive impairments linked to depression and schizophrenia and had poorer treatment outcomes. Quite the reverse, people with higher gray matter volume had a better prognosis of recovery from their mental illness. Based on this, increasing brain gray volume matter is important to achieve a positive outcome in youths with DMDD.

One potential supplement with promise to increase gray volume matter is fish oil, or more specifically, the polyunsaturated omega-3 essential fatty acids eicosapentaenoic acid (EPA) and docosahexaenoic acid (DHA) it contains. EPA and DHA are major structural lipid components of neural membranes that the brain relies upon for healthy structure and function. DHA is the most abundant omega-3 in gray matter. DHA is vital during infancy, childhood, and adolescence because these are periods of rapid gray matter expansion, neuronal maturation—when the nervous system connects and shapes brain circuitry to keep it functional, and formation of synapses between neurons. While

DHA can be created by the body from its fatty acid precursors, this process is inefficient, making supplementation crucial. EPA and DHA levels in the blood (red blood cell membranes) are measured via the Omega-3 Index. Optimally, one should score between 8 percent and 11 percent—though humans typically fall within the range of 2 to 20 percent—for a reduced risk of adverse health outcomes, including mental illness.[167] A typical Western diet, or the standard American diet (SAD), provide insufficient levels of EPA and DHA, thus necessitating supplementation.

A study evaluated the effects of dietary intake of EPA and DHA on gray matter volume in elderly individuals. The researchers found that those reporting eating more EPA- and DHA-rich foods had higher gray matter volume and improved cognitive performance.[168] Based on preclinical research showing that raising omega-3 fatty acids leads to structural brain changes, researchers assessed how omega-3s would affect human brain structure and function. Fifty-five healthy adults were evaluated for their average intake of omega-3s, and their brain gray matter was calculated by high-resolution structural MRI.[169] Participants who consumed higher levels of omega-3s had higher gray matter volume in areas of the brain associated with emotional arousal and regulation—bilateral anterior cingulate cortex, the right amygdala, and the right hippocampus—when compared to those who consumed less omega-3s. Mood was assessed in a separate study. People with higher blood levels of omega-3s had more agreeable moods and were less likely to report mild or moderate symptoms of depression. Conversely, people with low blood levels tended to have a negative outlook and be more impulsive. A systemic review and meta-analysis concluded that supplementation with EPA and DHA improves clinical symptoms of ADHD, and that deficiencies in omega-3s are common in children and youth with ADHD.[170] The totality of this evidence suggests that higher intake of EPA and DHA may promote structural and functional changes that lead to improved emotional and behavioral regulation.

Molecularly Distilled Fish Oil
_____

Typical dose: Dose providing ≥ 500 mg of DHA and EPA each, once or twice daily at mealtimes; in triglyceride—not ethyl ester—form

Contraindications: None currently known

Ask your health-care professional or pharmacist before using: Bipolar disorder, liver cirrhosis, diabetes, familial adenomatous polyposis, immunodeficiency, implantable defibrillators, seafood allergy

Potential interactions: Anticoagulant/antiplatelet drugs, blood pressure-lowering drugs, contraceptives, cyclosporine, orlistat, sirolimus; anticoagulant/antiplatelet supplements, supplements that lower blood pressure, fish oil may increase vitamin D and decrease vitamin E levels

Reported adverse effects: Abdominal pain, fishy aftertaste, heartburn, bad breath, increased low-density lipoprotein (LDL) cholesterol levels, loose stools, nausea, and rash

The other brain structural deficit that needs to be addressed in children with DMDD is brain cortical thickness. As described earlier, inadequate cortical thickness is associated with DMDD and other mental and behavioral disorders. Fortunately, a widely available and inexpensive supplement is available that may help. Vitamin D intake in the form of supplements has been associated with improved cortical thickness in humans.[171,172] Technically a steroid and not a vitamin, vitamin D is critical to brain health.

Vitamin D3
_____

Typical dose: Based on vitamin D levels, but somewhere in the range of 400–1,000 IU/day children aged six to ten; 800–4,000 IU/day children aged eleven to fourteen; and 3,000–10,000 IU/day for children aged fifteen to seventeen; your child's health-care professional may prescribe much higher doses in the case of vitamin D deficiency

Contraindications: Kidney disease

Ask your health-care professional or pharmacist before using: Arteriosclerosis, histoplasmosis, hypercalcemia, lymphoma, sarcoidosis, tuberculosis

Potential interactions: Aluminum, atorvastatin, calcipotriene, drugs metabolized by CYP3A4, digoxin, diltiazem, thiazide diuretics, verapamil; calcium and magnesium (vitamin D increases absorption of calcium and magnesium)

Reported adverse effects: Orally, vitamin D is well tolerated with few adverse effects reported

DETOXIFYING HEAVY METALS

As mentioned previously, heavy metals can interfere with nervous system function and contribute to mental illness and behavioral problems. Having small amounts of heavy metals like iron and copper is essential for healthy biological process, but storing large amounts can be toxic. Firstly, exposure to heavy metals should be minimized as much as possible. Filter drinking and bathing water. Don't use aluminum pans for cooking. Choose organic chicken and beef. Limit brown and white rice sourced from India where it tends to be higher in arsenic. Rice grown in California may be a better choice for its low arsenic content. Rinse rice before cooking and cook it using a six-to-one ratio of water to rice, draining off any leftover water. If you eat seafood, choose varieties that are low in mercury like wild-caught Alaskan salmon, pole-caught albacore tuna, and wild-caught Pacific sardines. Fish higher in mercury include Atlantic cod, shark, halibut, and swordfish. Use aluminum-free baking soda. Consider the vaccinations your children are receiving and how much aluminum and mercury they contain. Avoid mercury dental amalgams. Complete avoidance of heavy metals is impractical, but limiting exposure can go a long way in decreasing your child's toxic load and heavy metal body burden.

The human body is designed with amazingly complex systems to metabolize and eliminate heavy metals after they enter the body. Three primary mechanisms are used to do so: glutathione, metallothioneins, and porphyrins. A sulfur-containing tripeptide antioxidant, glutathione is produced within virtually all cells in the body. It has a remarkable metal-binding capacity, which helps the body eliminate toxic metals like mercury, arsenic, and lead. Glutathione production and function is dependent on adequate levels of B vitamins (B6 is very important to reduce lead accumulation in the body), sulfur, and selenium. Metallothioneins are also sulfur-containing, metal-biding proteins produced by many cells in the body. The production of metallothioneins is activated when the presence of heavy metals is detected. Their production is heavily reliant on sufficient protein and sulfur. Lastly, porphyrins do not contain sulfur but still have metal-binding capacity. Together, these three regulatory systems work to bind to and remove heavy metals and allow binding space for the smaller amounts of metals and elements necessary for healthy cellular function. Some of them pull heavy metals out of the cells, while others transport the heavy metals through the bloodstream or to the liver, gallbladder, kidneys, and intestines, where they can be eliminated.

A healthy gut lining is extremely important so that metals don't escape the intestinal tract and get back into the bloodstream. So, the leaky gut strategies also help with heavy metal detoxification. Supplementing with glutathione can provide more of this important antioxidant to handle heavy metal accumulation in cells. Moreover, providing dietary sulfur to produce glutathione and metallothioneins or adding sulfur-containing dietary supplements in the form of NAC, alpha-lipoic acid, and methylsulfonylmethane (MSM) may also aid heavy metal detoxification.

The symptoms of heavy metal toxicities may be an outward manifestation of a mineral deficiency. The body's heavy metal elimination mechanisms above can bind to essential elements and steal important minerals—zinc, magnesium, chromium, iron, molybdenum, selenium, and copper—from the body. Iron and zinc compete with heavy metals for intestinal absorption. Provide the body with ample amounts of minerals identified as insufficient or deficient in a mineral panel test.

We have multiple elimination channels—liver, bowel, kidneys, lungs, lymphatic system, blood, and skin—to handle toxins, including heavy metals. If these channels aren't working efficiently, waste and toxins start to recirculate, which can cause symptoms such as constipation, bloating, acne, respiratory issues, fatigue, sore muscles, and more. Providing foundational support for the body's natural elimination channels is essential. Elimination and detoxification should be personalized for the challenges an individual is facing, but should generally begin with a bowel cleanse so anything detoxified through other elimination channels doesn't end up relocating to the bowel. See a holistic health-care professional for a customized detoxification and elimination program.

LACTOBACILLUS PROBIOTICS

Before we leave the topic of heavy metals, it is worthwhile to mention the role of specific probiotic strains in heavy metal detoxification. Certain probiotics can bind to heavy metals, actively detoxify metals, and prevent the uptake of metals from the gastrointestinal tract.[173,174,175] Two of these strains include *Lactobacillus plantarum* CCFM8661 and *Lactobacillus rhamnosus* GR-1. These two strains represent an affordable way to counter exposures to toxic metals. Another strain, *Lactobacillus fermentum* ME-3, contains both glutathione peroxidase and glutathione reductase and can create glutathione, suggesting it can support the body's glutathione system.[176] Quite simply, probiotics are one of the greatest keys to health and their wide-ranging biological properties make them essential dietary supplements.

Lactobacillus rhamnosus, L. plantarum, and *L. fermentum* ME-3

Typical dose: 10 billion CFU daily

Contraindications: Serious immunosuppression

Ask your health-care professional or pharmacist before using: Pancreatitis

Potential interactions: Should be taken at least two to four hours after antibiotics or antifungals

Reported adverse effects: Digestive upset

ESSENTIAL OILS

Essential oils are volatile organic compounds extracted from plants. They act as small facilitative messenger molecules that help to heal, protect, and guide cells. By doing so, they make body systems work better, and the whole person can thrive. One great property of essential oils is that their molecular weight enables them to readily cross the blood-brain barrier and enter brain tissues.[177,178,179] Once there, they may enhance cerebral blood flow, bind to receptors, promote the release of neurochemicals, and stimulate neuroendocrine responses. One of the fastest ways for essential oils to influence nervous system function is through inhalation because of their access to the brain.

Preclinical research suggests that lemon essential oil influences the release of both serotonin and dopamine, particularly increasing dopamine in the prefrontal cortex and hippocampus.[180] Clove essential oil may restore dopamine function by increasing dopamine transporter (DAT) activity.[181] DAT is a protein that is responsible for the reuptake of dopamine and a major target of stimulant drugs like methylphenidate

(methylphenidate and other stimulants interfere with its activity). Other essential oils may trigger changes in brainwave activity.[182] The formation of neurites (neuritogenesis) is a fundamental process in the developing nervous system that builds a complex communication network of neurons. The primary constituent of copaiba (*Copaifera* spp.) essential oil, beta-caryophyllene, promotes neuritogenesis and as a side benefit reduces inflammation and protects nervous system structure and function.[183,184] Aromatherapy is a non-invasive and highly effective tool to support balanced brain activity and potentially reduce the symptoms of DMDD.

Create a diffuser blend with the following essential oils and diffuse while sleeping and when your child will remain in the same room with the diffuser for at least thirty minutes:

- 4 drops of lemon
- 2 drops of clove
- 2 drops of copaiba
- 1 drop of black pepper

Create a topical-roller-bottle blend in a 10 mL roller bottle as below and apply topically to the back of the neck and temples at least twice daily:

- 5 drops of copaiba
- 3 drops of frankincense
- 2 drops of black pepper
- 2 drops of vetiver
- 2 drops of lavender
- 1 drop of clove bud
- 1 drop ylang ylang

Natural solutions are regulated in the United States by the FDA, but not approved like drugs. Pharmaceuticals have their place in integrative medicine, and there are cases in which a drug is necessary to save life or improve life quality. Additionally, modern medicine has made it possible to extend life with remarkable surgeries like organ transplants. However, there are just as many cases where a natural solution or therapy can be beneficial without the harmful side effects associated with many medications and surgeries. Natural remedies have been used for centuries, and in many cases millennia, to help the body perform its primary duty to defend itself and maintain a state of health. The goal is to use the least invasive and least dangerous solution that is still effective.

Contrary to drugs, natural solutions seek to promote healthy function of various systems in the body innately present to maintain a state of health. They do so by working with the body's corrective actions, removing roadblocks that hinder health restoration, and aiding cells, organs, and organ systems in their healthy functions. They do not mask symptoms but go deeper to address the root cause of the problem. Countless studies demonstrate their effectiveness and safety for a variety of conditions. Moreover, while drugs rely upon a single (possibly two) active molecules, herbs and essential oils are natural complex substances with multiple compounds that can provide additive, synergistic, and antagonistic actions within a single herb or essential oil. The effectiveness and usefulness of natural remedies has thousands of years of use compared to mere hundreds for chemical medicines. Many people are reconnecting with the healing power of our nature that our ancestors relied upon to enjoy greater wellness naturally.

4

....

LIFESTYLE ADJUSTMENTS

Lifestyle changes are simple but powerful tools to address mood and behavioral disorders. Sometimes lifestyle changes alone can significantly reduce symptoms, making it important to not overlook this as a strategy for your child with DMDD. Taking a greater control over his lifestyle, thoughts, and behaviors leads to a better chance of managing DMDD more effectively. Lifestyle adjustments can turn the tides in your favor and help your child feel better, which encourages even more progress.

NUTRITION

Nutrition is the foundation of wellness. You are what you eat is quite literal because food and beverages are broken down into smaller molecules that are then incorporated into tissues. Eating more nutritious foods—more vegetables and fruits, legumes, nuts, high quality protein, and whole grains—has been consistently correlated with a decreased risk of mood disorders.[185] Conversely, the Western diet has been repeatedly linked to an increased risk of mood disorders. Dietary modifications are a foundational step to managing DMDD.

Better quality nutrition has been associated with larger brain volumes, including gray matter volume.[186] This study evaluated the diets of more than 4,200 individuals and performed brain MRIs to assess the participant's brain tissue volumes. What the researchers found was that people who ate more vegetables, fruit, whole grains, nuts, dairy, and fish and fewer sugary beverages had larger brain volumes. Specifically, they had larger gray matter volume, white matter volume, and hippocampal volume. Another smaller study reported that people who consumed more alcohol and animal foods had lower brain gray matter volume.[187] Surprisingly, consuming more milk and yogurt promoted a normal volume of gray matter. The evidence suggests that nutrition can directly affect the structure and therefore function of the brain.

Eating anti-inflammatory foods can also influence brain gray matter volumes. Inflammation is a vital function controlled by the immune system that serves to protect against infection, illness, and injury. However, chronic inflammation in specific tissues or systemic inflammation can drive illnesses, including mental illnesses. As part of the inflammatory process, the immune system releases antibodies to fight infection or repair the problem. A filter called the blood-brain barrier normally protects the brain from those antibodies. But if these antibodies cross the filter and enter brain tissues, they disrupt neurotransmitters, interfering with brain function.[188] Eating foods that provoke an inflammatory response in the body was correlated with smaller total brain volume and gray matter volume even after adjustment for demographic, clinical, and other lifestyle variables.[189] Pro-inflammatory foods and ingredients include sugar, high fructose corn syrup, fried foods, refined carbohydrates, processed foods, certain highly-refined seed and vegetable oils (e.g., corn, canola, and soy), alcohol in excess, and meats cooked at high temperatures. Rather than disrupting your child's diet overnight, start slowly by introducing or removing one food at a time.

The body relies on a steady stream of antioxidants from dietary sources, which reduce free radical levels in the body. Excess free radicals can increase inflammation. Vegetables and fruits usually have high levels of dietary antioxidants. Foods that should be incorporated into the diet to counteract inflammation include cruciferous vegetables, fruits (especially dark-colored fruits like blueberries, cherries, and grapes), high-fat fruits (avocados, olives), fatty fish, healthy oils (olive and avocado oil), nuts, dark chocolate, peppers, and spices (turmeric, cinnamon, fenugreek).

PHYSICAL ACTIVITY

It's not surprising that what is good for general health and well-being is also good to manage DMDD, and this includes movement and physical activity. We all know that regular physical activity keeps us physically healthy, but regular activity also makes your child feel good mentally and emotionally. Physical activity can boost mood, alertness, and concentration. Physical activity alters neurochemicals (like serotonin, dopamine, and norepinephrine) in the brain and releases feel-good chemicals called endorphins—natural brain chemicals that enhance the sense of well-being. Simultaneously, physical activity decreases levels of the stress hormone cortisol. Not to mention that physical activity can be a distraction from negative thoughts. Additionally, it reduces inflammation through several mechanisms, which improves outcomes for people experiencing a mood disorder.[190] Find a physical activity that your child enjoys and encourage them to participate in it regularly. If possible, make it a team or group activity that can provide social opportunities, chances to learn healthy ways to engage with peers, and learn teamwork.

ATTITUDE OF GRATITUDE

Encourage your child to adopt an attitude of gratitude and document what she is grateful for in a journal. More than a feeling of thankfulness, gratitude involves neuroscience and alterations in the brain that improve well-being. What your child's brain looks like on gratitude is best described as a neurochemical cocktail that includes serotonin and dopamine. When expressing gratitude, neural circuitry in the brain releases dopamine that makes one feel good. This may partly explain why serving others feels so good. Higher dopamine levels feels good, triggers positive emotions, and fosters greater optimism. To boost this effect, encourage your child to write down or seriously reflect on what she is grateful for. Doing so triggers her anterior cingulate cortex to release serotonin. Serotonin enhances mood, willpower, and motivation. Even better, the more these circuits of gratitude are activated, the stronger their corresponding neural pathways become and the more likely your child is to feel positive.

RESTORATIVE SLEEP

Inadequate or nonrestful sleep has a significant impact on mood. This may be where the term "woke up on the wrong side of the bed" comes from. Restorative sleep, which occurs during the third stage of non-REM sleep, is necessary to maintain balanced brain function and a healthy mood. Interestingly, people who don't get enough sleep each night have a greater tendency to classify neutral and pleasant images as negative—something already observed in youths with DMDD.[191] In other words, lack of sleep makes us view the world as more menacing, predisposing us to a negative mood.

Encourage your child to practice good sleep hygiene—fostering a bedroom environment and daily routines that promote, consistent uninterrupted sleep—practices, particularly at a young age. Getting your teen to implement these same habits can be very challenging given their irregular sleep patterns and constant screen time. The following sleep hygiene practices can not only reduce the symptoms of DMDD, but are important for physical, mental, and emotional health, and improve overall quality of life.

Strive to go to bed and wake up at the same time every day. An irregular sleep schedule can interfere with your child's circadian rhythm and reduce restful sleep. Maintain a consistent bedtime routine.

Cultivate healthy daily habits. Expose your child to regular sunlight, which promotes a healthy circadian rhythm. Encourage them to be physically active during the day. Seek to limit her caffeine consumption in the afternoon and evening. Discourage your child from watching television, scrolling mindlessly on her phone, and other activities outside of sleeping in her bed. This builds a link in her mind that a bed is for sleeping.

Prioritize sleep. Although your child may want to stay up late to binge-watch her favorite show, sleep must be a priority. Shortening sleep can disrupt mood and quality of life.

Optimize your child's bedroom environment. Make sure her room is dark—use blackout curtains if necessary. Ensure a comfortable room temperature, erring on the cooler side (near 65 degrees Fahrenheit). Invest in a comfortable mattress and pillow and choose sheets and blankets that your child prefers the texture of. Consider a weighted blanket.

Allow for a thirty-minute wind-down period before bed. Urge your child to stop screen exposure—which exposes him to blue light that can disrupt his circadian rhythm—at least thirty minutes before bed. Instead, he should focus on calming music, reading, light stretching, or relaxation exercises.

Incorporate calming scents. Diffuse essential oils like lavender, chamomile, woodsy oils, or citruses beginning about thirty minutes prior to bed.

HEALTHY CONNECTIONS & RELATIONSHIPS

Every single person needs a friend or person they share a meaningful and authentic relationship with. Young children experience life through relationships, and the health of their relationships shapes nearly all aspects of their development. Children crave attention, whether positive or negative, because they thrive on it. Healthy relationships teach children how to behave, enhance self-confidence, and improve mental, emotional, and physical health.

Unhealthy relationships can cause a child to reflect and portray negative feelings in their other relationships, such as school and among their peers. Kids learn through what they observe from others, making modeling healthy relationships at home vital. Additionally, healthy relationships act as a source of love and support through difficult times.

Devote time and effort to building a positive relationship with your child. Set appropriate boundaries that build respect in the home. Look for shared interests. Engage in meaningful activities with her. Children want time with their parents. Providing your child with the opportunity to have a warm and positive relationship with you can improve your child's behavior and increase the likelihood of a positive outcome managing DMDD.

Strive to engage your child in clubs, sports, music, dance, or other extracurricular activities that give them opportunities to interact with other children their age. More exposure to peers gives them opportunities to form positive relationships, learn communication skills, interpret body language, and cooperate as part of a team. Having well-developed social skills leads to improved cognitive abilities and improves mental and emotional health.

Life with DMDD is complicated for the whole family. There will be times you feel you need to walk on eggshells to avoid an explosive outburst. Taking control of lifestyle factors that you can, and forgetting about what you can't, helps the whole family in dealing with this disorder.

5

HOPE TO BEAT DMDD

By now, you as the parent should have a lot of thoughts about what to do next. Don't try to execute everything at once. Instead, try one or two items at a time and take time to allow progress and changes to occur. Remember that natural solutions and lifestyle adjustments are not like drugs and normally don't have an immediate effect. Some of them can take several weeks to observe results. The key is to be consistent and patient, provide emotional support to your child, take care of your own mental health, and balance the needs of your child with DMDD while maintaining the needs of other family members. It's also very important to incorporate multiple strategies, especially therapy that helps your child interpret social interactions better and discover better ways to cope with frustration other than rage. Natural solutions are not a quick fix, but they are frequently the long-term fix your child needs.

It is essential that you find a mental health professional who is experienced with DMDD and a good fit for your child and family. Don't seek to manage DMDD all on your own. It will take an entire community of people to provide a safe and healthy environment for your child to grow and develop and learn to better cope with DMDD. Your entire family will be affected by DMDD, not just the child with it. Consequently, it makes sense to involve the whole family in better understanding the condition and appropriate ways to interact with the child with DMDD.

Parenting a child with DMDD is a difficult roller coaster that often makes parents feel paralyzed without direction or hope. DMDD is a silent condition that is not obvious to other parents and children, which can increase feelings of being alone in this battle. However, equipped with a better understanding of DMDD and your child as well as empowered with how to incorporate effective natural solutions, you can beat DMDD and get your son or daughter back. It doesn't mean that they will never be moody, irritable, or angry, but with patience and the implementation of the strategies in this book, you can have more positive days with your child and break the cycle of explosive confrontations. Impossible becomes *I'm possible* when you separate the *im* from the *possible*. Although daunting, you can succeed in being the super mom or dad your child with DMDD needs to transition into adulthood successfully!

REFERENCES

[1] American Academy of Pediatrics, American Academy of Child Adolescent Psychiatry, and Children's Hospital Association. AAP-AACAP-CHA Declaration of a National Emergency in Child and Adolescent Mental Health. Available at: https://www.aap.org/en/advocacy/child-and-adolescent-healthy-mental-development/aap-aacap-cha-declaration-of-a-national-emergency-in-child-and-adolescent-mental-health/. Accessed January 4, 2023.

[2] National Institute of Mental Health. Disruptive Mood Dysregulation Disorder: The Basics. Available at: https://www.nimh.nih.gov/health/publications/disruptive-mood-dysregulation-disorder. Accessed January 4, 2022.

[3] Copeland WE, Angold A, Costello EJ, et al. Prevalence, comorbidity, and correlates of DSM-5 proposed disruptive mood dysregulation disorder. *Am J Psychiatry*. 2013 Feb;170(2):173-9.

[4] Copeland WE, Angold A, Costello EJ, et al. Prevalence, comorbidity, and correlates of DSM-5 proposed disruptive mood dysregulation disorder. *Am J Psychiatry*. 2013 Feb;170(2):173-9.

[5] Grau K, Plener PL, Hohmann S, et al. Prevalence Rate and Course of Symptoms of Disruptive Mood Dysregulation Disorder (DMDD). *Zeitschrift für Kinder- und Jugendpsychiatrie und Psychotherapie*. 2018;46(1):29-38.

[6] Mrockzkowski MM, McReynolds LS, Fisher P, et al. Disruptive Mood Dysregulation Disorder in Juvenile Justice. *J Am Academy Psych Law*. 2018 Sep;46(3):329-38.

[7] Blok E, White T. Editorial: White Matter Matters: Neurobiological Differences Between Pediatric Bipolar Disorder and Disruptive Mood Dysregulation Disorder. *J Am Acad Child Adolesc Psychiatry*. 2020 Oct;59(10):1128-1129.

[8] Masi L, Gignac M. ADHD and DMDD comorbidities, similarities and distinctions. *J Child Adolesc Behav*. 2016;4(6):1000325.

[9] Dickstein DP, Rich BA, Binstock AB, et al. Comorbid Anxiety in Phenotypes of Pediatric Bipolar Disorder. *J Child Adolesc Psychopharm*. 2005 Aug;15(4):534-48.

[10] Axelson D, Findling RL, Fristad MA, et al. Examining the proposed disruptive mood dysregulation disorder diagnosis in children in the Longitudinal Assessment of Manic Symptoms study. *J Clin Psychiatry*. 2012;73:1342–50.

[11] Starr R, MacLean D, Keating D. (1991). Life-Span Development of Child Maltreatment: The Effects of Child Abuse and Neglect. New York, NY: The Guilford Press.

[12] Wolfe D, McGree R. (1991). Assessment of Emotional Status Among Maltreated Children: The Effects of Child Abuse and Neglect. New York, NY: The Guilford Press.

[13] Benarous X, Renaud J, Breton JJ, et al. Are youths with disruptive mood dysregulation disorder different from youths with major depressive disorder or persistent depressive disorder? *J Affective Disorders*. 2020 Mar 15;265:207-15.

[14] Jaworska-Andryszewska P, Rybakowski JK. Childhood trauma in mood disorders: Neurobiological mechanisms and implications for treatment. *Pharmacol Rep*. 2019 Feb;71(1):112-120.

[15] Liu J, Raine A, Venables PH, et al. Malnutrition at age 3 years and externalizing behavior problems at ages 8, 11, and 17 years. *Am J Psychiatry*. 2004 Nov;161(11):2005-13.

[16] Gelenberg AJ. Psychiatric Disorders, in DM Paige, Ed. Clinical Nutrition, Second Edition. St. Louis, The C.V. Mosby Company, 1988.

[17] Hodges RE, Bean WB, Ohlson MA, et al. Human pantothenic acid deficiency produced by omega-methyl pantothenic acid. *J Clin Invest*. 1959;38(8):1421-25.

[18] Lonsdale D, Shamberger RJ. Red cell transketolase as an indicator of nutritional deficiency. *Am J Clin Nutr*. 1980 Feb;33(2):205-11.

[19] McLaren DS. Clinical manifestations of nutritional disorders, in ME Shils & VR Young. Modern Nutrition in Health and Disease, Seventh Edition. Philadelphia, Lea & Febiger, 1988.

[20] Wilmot CA, et al. Ascorbic acid inhibits isolation-induced fighting in mice. *Fed Proc*. 1983;42:1160.

[21] Robinson SL, Marín C, Oliveros H, et al. Vitamin D deficiency in middle childhood is related to behavior problems in adolescence. *J Nutr*. 2020 Jan 1;150(1):140-148.

[22] Bahrami A, Mazloum SR, Maghsoudi S, et al. High Dose Vitamin D Supplementation Is Associated With a Reduction in Depression Score Among Adolescent Girls: A Nine-Week Follow-Up Study. *J Diet Suppl*. 2018 Mar 4;15(2):173-182.

[23] Youdim MB, Ben-Shachar D, Yehuda S. Putative biological mechanisms of the effect of iron deficiency on brain biochemistry and behavior. *Am J Clin Nutr*. 1989 Sep;50(3 Suppl):607-15.

[24] Webb TE, Oski FA. Behavioral Status of Young Adolescents with Iron Deficiency Anemia. *J Special Ed*. 1974;8(2):153-6.

[25] Kantak KM. Magnesium deficiency alters aggressive behavior and catecholamine function. *Behav Neurosci*. 1988 Apr;102(2):304-11.

[26] Mousain-Bose M, Roche M, Rapin J, et al. Magnesium VitB6 Intake Reduces Central Nervous System Hyperexcitability in Children. *J Am Coll Nutr*. 2004 Oct;23(5):545S-548S.

[27] Roy A, Virkkunen M, Linnoila M. Monamines, glucose metabolism, aggression towards self and others. *Int J Neurosci*. 1988 Aug;41(3-4):261-4.

[28] Linnoila VM, Virkkunen M. Aggression, suicidality, and serotonin. *J Clin Psychiatry*. 1992 Oct;53 Suppl:46-51.

[29] Ferro MA, Lieshout RJV, Ohayon J, et al. Emotional and behavioral problems in adolescents and young adults with food allergy. *Allergy*. 2016 Apr;71(4):532-40.

[30] Hart GR. Food-Specific IgG Guided Elimination Diet; A Role in Mental Health? *BAOJ Nut*. 2017;3(1):045.

[31] Hofeldt FD. Reactive hypoglycemia. *Endocrinol Metab Clin North Am*. 1989 Mar;18(1):185-201.

[32] Matijasevich A, Murray J, Cooper P, et al. Trajectories of maternal depression and offspring psychopathology at 6 years: Pelotas cohort study. *J Affective Disorders*. 2015;174:424–431.

[33] Hope S, Pearce A, Chittleborough C, et al. Temporal effects of maternal psychological distress on child mental health problems at ages 3, 5, 7 and 11: analysis from the UK Millennium Cohort Study. *Psychol Med*. 2019 Mar;49(4):664–674.

[34] Wolicki SB, Bitsko RH, Cree RA, et al. Mental Health of Parents and Primary Caregivers by Sex and Associated Child Health Indicators. *Adversity Resilience Sci*. 2021;2:125–139.

[35] Singleton L. Parental mental illness: the effects on children and their needs. *Br J Nurs*. 2007;16(14):847-50.

[36] Thomson GO, Raab GM, Hepburn WS, et al. Blood-lead levels and children's behaviour--results from the Edinburgh Lead Study. *J Child Psychol Psychiatry*. 1989 Jul;30(4):515-28.

[37] Klotz K, Weisterhofer W, Neff F, et al. The Health Effects of Aluminum Exposure. *Dtsch Arztebl Int*. 2017 Sep;114(39):653–659.

[38] Pearson H. Mercury affects brains of adolescents. *Nature*. 200 Feb 64:422.

[39] Patel NB, Xu Y, McCandless LC, et al. Very low-level prenatal mercury exposure and behaviors in children: the HOME Study. *Environ Health*. 2019 Jan 9;18(1):4.

[40] Gump BB, Dykas MJ, MacKenzie JA, et al. Background lead and mercury exposures: Psychological and behavioral problems in children. *Environ Res*. 2017 Oct;158:576-582.

[41] Nowak G, Szewczyk B, Pilc A. Zinc and depression. An update. *Pharmacol Reports*. 2005;57:713-18.

[42] Petrilli MA, Kranz TM, Kleinhaus K, et al. The Emerging Role for Zinc in Depression and Psychosis. *Front Pharmacol*. 2017;8:414.

[43] Royer A, Sharman T. Copper Toxicity. Available at: https://www.ncbi.nlm.nih.gov/books/NBK557456/. Accessed January 6, 2023.

[44] Martinez EJ, Kolb BL, Bell A, et al. Moderate perinatal arsenic exposure alters neuroendocrine markers associated with depression and increases depressive-like behaviors in adult mouse offspring. *Neurotoxicol.* 2008;29(4):647–655.

[45] Syed EH, Poudel KC, Sakisaka K, et al. Quality of life and mental health status of arsenic-affected patients in a Bangladeshi population. *J Health Popul Nutr.* 2012 Sep;30(3):262-9.

[46] Tolins M, Ruchirawat M, Landrigan P. The developmental neurotoxicity of arsenic: cognitive and behavioral consequences of early life exposure. *Ann Glob Health.* 2014 Jul-Aug;80(4):303-14.

[47] Tseng WL, Deveney CM, Stoddard J, et al. Brain Mechanisms of Attention Orienting Following Frustration: Associations With Irritability and Age in Youths. *Am J Psychiatry.* 2019 Jan 1;176(1):67-76.

[48] Seok JW, Bajaj S, Soltis-Vaughan B, et al. Structural atrophy of the right superior frontal gyrus in adolescents with severe irritability. *Hum Brain Mapp.* 2021 Oct 1;42(14):4611-4622.

[49] Zhang X, Yao S, Zhu X, et al. Gray matter volume abnormalities in individuals with cognitive vulnerability to depression: a voxel-based morphometry study. *J Affect Disord.* 2012 Feb;136(3):443-52.

[50] Zhao Y, Chen L, Zhang W, et al. Gray Matter Abnormalities in Non-comorbid Medication-naive Patients with Major Depressive Disorder or Social Anxiety Disorder. *EBioMedicine.* 2017 Jul;21:228-235.

[51] Bonath B, Tegelbeckers J, Wilke M, et al. Regional Gray Matter Volume Differences Between Adolescents With ADHD and Typically Developing Controls: Further Evidence for Anterior Cingulate Involvement. *J Atten Disord.* 2018 May;22(7):627-638.

[52] Li L, Zuo Y, Chen Y. Relationship between local gyrification index and age, intelligence quotient, symptom severity with Autism Spectrum Disorder: A large-scale MRI study. *J Clin Neurosci.* 2021 Sep;91:193-199.

[53] Gharegazlou A, Vandewouw M, Ziolowski J, et al. Cortical Gyrification Morphology in ASD and ADHD: Implication for Further Similarities or Disorder-Specific Features? *Cereb Cortex.* 2022 May 30;32(11):2332-2342.

[54] Long J, Xu J, Wang X, et al. Altered Local Gyrification Index and Corresponding Functional Connectivity in Medication Free Major Depressive Disorder.*front Psychiatry.* 2020 dec 14;11:585401.

[55] Leibenluft E, Stoddard J. The developmental psychopathology of irritability. *Dev Psychopathol.* 2013;25(4 Pt 2):1473–1487.

[56] Leibenluft E. Severe mood dysregulation, irritability, and the diagnostic boundaries of bipolar disorder in youths. *Am J Psychiatry.* 2011;168(2):129–142.

[57] Stoddard J, Sharif-Askay B, Harkins EA, et al. An Open Pilot Study of Training Hostile Interpretation Bias to Treat Disruptive Mood Dysregulation Disorder. *J Child Adolesc Psychopharmacol.* 2016 Feb 1;26(1):49–57.

[58] Thomas L, Kim P, Bones B, et al. Elevated amygdala responses to emotional faces in youths with chronic irritability or bipolar disorder. *NeuroImage Clin.* 2013;2:637–645.

[59] Brotman M, Rich B, Guyer A, et al. Amygdala activation during emotion processing of neutral faces in children with severe mood dysregulation versus ADHD or bipolar disorder. *Am J Psych.* 2010;167(1):61–69.

[60] Stoddard J, Tseng W, Kim P, et al. Association of irritability and anxiety with the neural mechanisms of implicit face emotion processing in youths with psychopathology. *JAMA Psych.* 2017;74(1):95.

[61] Kircanski K, White L, Tseng WL, et al. A Latent variable approach to differentiating neural mechanisms of irritability and anxiety in youth. *JAMA Psych.* 2018;75(6):631.

[62] Benarous X, Bury V, Lahyae H, et al. Sensory Processing Difficulties in Youths With Disruptive Mood Dysregulation Disorder. *Front Psychiatry.* 2020 Mar 23;11:164.

[63] Roberson-Nay R, Leibenluft E, Brotman MA, et al. Longitudinal Stability of Genetic and Environmental Influences on Irritability: From Childhood to Young Adulthood. *Am J Psych.* 2015;172(7):657–664.

[64] Moore AA, Lapato DM, Botman MA, et al. Heritability, stability, and prevalence of tonic and phasic irritability as indicators of Disruptive Mood Dysregulation Disorder. *J Child Psychol Psychiatry.* 2019 Sep;60(9):1032–1041.

[65] O'Leary III JC, Zhang B, Korn III J, et al. The role of FKBP5 in mood disorders: Action of FKBP5 on steroid hormone receptors leads to questions about its evolutionary importance. *CNS Neurol Disord Drug Targets.* 2013 Dec;12(8):1157–1162.

[66] Dixit A, Mahour P, Agarwal V. Cognitive Behavioural Therapy for Disruptive Mood Dysregulation Disorder. *Indian J Mental Health.* 2020;7(2):158-162.

[67] Tudor ME, Ibrahim K, Bertschinger E, et al. Cognitive-Behavioral Therapy for a 9-Year-Old Girl With Disruptive Mood Dysregulation Disorder. *Clin Case Stud.* 2016 Dec;15(6):459–475.

[68] Linke J, Kircanski K, Brooks J, et al. Exposure-Based Cognitive-Behavioral Therapy for Disruptive Mood Dysregulation Disorder: An Evidence-Based Case Study. *Behav Ther.* 2020 Mar;51(2):320-333.

[69] Waxomonsky JG, Wymbs FA, Pariseau ME, et al. A Novel Group Therapy for Children With ADHD and Severe Mood Dysregulation. *J Atten Disord*. 2013;17(6):527–541.

[70] Stoddard J, Sharif-Askary B, Harkins EA, et al. An Open Pilot Study of Training Hostile Interpretation Bias to Treat Disruptive Mood Dysregulation Disorder. *J Child Adolesc Psychopharmacol*. 2016 Feb;26(1):49-57.

[71] Stoddard J, Sharif-Askary B, Harkins EA, et al. An open pilot study of training hostile interpretation bias to treat disruptive mood dysregulation disorder. *J Child Adolesc Psychopharmacol*. 2016;26(1):49–57.

[72] Baweja R, Belin PJ, Humphrey HH, et al. The effectiveness and tolerability of central nervous system stimulants in school-age children with attention-deficit/hyperactivity disorder and disruptive mood dysregulation disorder across home and school. *J Child Adolesc Psychopharmacol*. 2016 Mar;26(2):154-63.

[73] Winters DE, Fukui S, Leibenluft E, et al. Improvements in Irritability with Open-Label Methylphenidate Treatment in Youth with Comorbid Attention Deficit/Hyperactivity Disorder and Disruptive Mood Dysregulation Disorder. *J Child Adolesc Psychopharmacol*. 2018 Jun;28(5):298-305.

[74] Jain U. The use of guanfacine (Intuniv XR) in the treatment of disruptive mood dysregulation disorder – Clinical experience from telepsychiatry. *Eur Psych*. 2017 Apr;41(S1):S442.

[75] Carminati GG, Gerber F, Darbellay B, et al. Using venlafaxine to treat behavioral disorders in patients with autism spectrum disorder. *Prog Neuropsychopharmacol Biol Psychiatry*. 2016 Feb 4;65:85-95.

[76] Pappadopulos E, Woolston S, Chait A, et al. Pharmacotherapy of Aggression in Children and Adolescents: Efficacy and Effect Size. *J Can Acad Child Adolesc Psychiatry*. 2006 Feb; 15(1): 27–39.

[77] McGough J. Characterization and Sequential Pharmacotherapy of Severe Mood Dysregulation. Available at: https://clinicaltrials.gov/ct2/show/NCT01714310. Accessed January 4, 2023.

[78] Pappadopulos E, Woolston S, Chait A, et al. Pharmacotherapy of Aggression in Children and Adolescents: Efficacy and Effect Size. *J Can Acad Child Adolesc Psychiatry*. 2006 Feb; 15(1): 27–39.

[79] Tiihonen J, Lehti M, Aaltonen, et al. Psychotropic drugs and homicide: a prospective cohort study from Finland. *World Psych*. 2015 Jun;14(2):245-7.

[80] Moore TJ, Glenmullen J, Furberg CD. Prescription drugs associated with reports of violence towards others. *PLoS One*. 2010 Dec 15;5(12):e15337.

[81] Pappadopulos E, Woolston S, Chait A, et al. Pharmacotherapy of Aggression in Children and Adolescents: Efficacy and Effect Size. *J Can Acad Child Adolesc Psychiatry*. 2006 Feb; 15(1): 27–39.

[82] Pappadopulos E, Woolston S, Chait A, et al. Pharmacotherapy of Aggression in Children and Adolescents: Efficacy and Effect Size. *J Can Acad Child Adolesc Psychiatry*. 2006 Feb; 15(1): 27–39.

[83] Biederman J, Baldessarini RJ, Wright V, et al. A double-blind placebo controlled study of desipramine in the treatment of ADD: I. efficacy. *J Am Acad Child Adolesc Psychiatry*. 1989 Sep;28(5):777-84.

[84] Krieger FV, Pheula GF, Coelho R, Zeni T, et al. An open-label trial of risperidone in children and adolescents with severe mood dysregulation. *J Child Adolesc Psychopharmacol*. 2011 Jun;21(3):237-43.

[85] Aman MG, Bukstein OG, Gadow KD, et al. What does risperidone add to parent training and stimulant for severe aggression in child attention-deficit/hyperactivity disorder? *J Am Acad Child Adolesc Psychiatry*. 2014 Jan;53(1):47-60.

[86] Zeni CP, Tramontina S, Ketzer CR, et al. Methylphenidate combined with aripiprazole in children and adolescents with bipolar disorder and attention-deficit/hyperactivity disorder: a randomized crossover trial. *J Child Adolesc Psychopharmacol*. 2009 Oct;19(5):553-61.

[87] Pan PY, Fu AT, Yeh CB. Aripiprazole/Methylphenidate Combination in Children and Adolescents with Disruptive Mood Dysregulation Disorder and Attention-Deficit/Hyperactivity Disorder: An Open-Label Study. *J Child Adolesc Psychopharmacol*. 2018 Dec;28(10):682-689.

[88] Findling RL, Mankoski R, Timko K, et al. A randomized controlled trial investigating the safety and efficacy of aripiprazole in the long-term maintenance treatment of pediatric patients with irritability associated with autistic disorder. *J Clin Psych*. 2014;75(1):22–30.

[89] Cohen D, Raffin M, Canitano R, et al. Risperidone or aripiprazole in children and adolescents with autism and/or intellectual disability: A Bayesian meta-analysis of efficacy and secondary effects. *Res Autism Spectrum Disorders*. 2013;7(1):167–175.

[90] Aman MG, Binder C, Turgay A. Risperidone effects in the presence/absence of psychostimulant medicine in children with ADHD, other disruptive behavior disorders, and subaverage IQ. J Child Adolescent Psychopharm. 2004;14(2):243–254.

[91] Connor DF, McLaughlin TJ, Jeffers-Terry M. Randomized controlled pilot study of quetiapine in the treatment of adolescent conduct disorder. *J Child Adolesc Psychopharm*. 2008;18(2):140–156

[92] Anderson LT, Campbell M, Adams P, et al. The effects of haloperidol on discrimination learning and behavioral symptoms in autistic children. *J Autism Develop Disorders*. 1989;19(2):227–239.

[93] Campbell M, Small AM, Green WH, et al. Behavioral efficacy of haloperidol and lithium carbonate. A comparison in hospitalized aggressive children with conduct disorder. *Arch Gen Psych*. 1984;41(7):650–656.

[94] Hellings JA, Weckbaugh M, Nickel EJ, et al. A double-blind, placebo-controlled study of valproate for aggression in youth with pervasive developmental disorders. *J Child Adolesc Psychopharm*. 2005;15(4):682–692.

[95] Donovan SJ, Stewart JW, Nunes EV, et al. Divalproex treatment for youth with explosive temper and mood lability: A double-blind, placebo-controlled crossover design. *Am J Psych*. 2000;157(5):818–820.

[96] Hollander E, Chaplin W, Soorya L, et al. Divalproex sodium vs placebo for the treatment of irritability in children and adolescents with autism spectrum disorders. *Neuropsychopharmacology*. 2009;35(4):990–998.

[97] Belsito KM, Law PA, Kirk KS, et al. Lamotrigine therapy for autistic disorder: A randomized, double-blind, placebo-controlled trial. *J Autism Development Disorders*. 2001;31(2):175–181.

[98] Cueva JE, Overall JE, Small AM, et al. Carbamazepine in aggressive children with conduct disorder: A double-blind and placebo-controlled study. *J Am Academy Child Adolesc Psych*. 1996;35(4):480–490.

[99] National Alliance for Mental Illness (NAMI). Valproate (Depakote). Available at: https://nami.org/About-Mental-Illness/Treatments/Mental-Health-Medications/Types-of-Medication/Valproate-(Depakote). Accessed January 5, 2023.

[100] Dickstein DP, Towbin KE, Van Der Veen JW, et al. Randomized double-blind placebo-controlled trial of lithium in youth with severe mood dysregulation. *J Child Adolesc Psychopharmacol*. 2009;19:61–73.

[101] de la Cruz LF, Simonoff E, McGough JJ, et al. Treatment of children with attention-deficit/hyperactivity disorder (ADHD) and irritability: Results from the multimodal treatment study of children with ADHD (MTA). *J Am Acad Child Adolesc Psychiatry*. 2015;54:62–70.

[102] Tourian L, LeBoeuf A, Breton JJ, et al. Treatment options for the cardinal symptoms of disruptive mood dysregulation disorder. *J Can Acad Child Adolesc Psychiatry*. 2015;24:41–54.

[103] de la Cruz LF, Simonoff E, McGough JJ, et al. Treatment of children with attention-deficit/hyperactivity disorder (ADHD) and irritability: Results from the multimodal treatment study of children with ADHD (MTA). *J Am Acad Child Adolesc Psychiatry*. 2015;54:62–70.

[104] Parmar A, Vats D, Parmar R, et al. Role of naltrexone in management of behavioral outbursts in an adolescent male diagnosed with disruptive mood dysregulation disorder. *J Child Adolesc Psychopharmacol*. 2014;24(10):594–595.

[105] Pappadopulos E, Woolston S, Chait A, et al. Pharmacotherapy of Aggression in Children and Adolescents: Efficacy and Effect Size. *J Can Acad Child Adolesc Psychiatry*. 2006 Feb; 15(1): 27–39.

[106] Chatterjee M, Verma R, Kimari R, et al. Antipsychotic activity of standardized Bacopa extract against ketamine-induced experimental psychosis in mice: Evidence for the involvement of dopaminergic, serotonergic, and cholinergic systems. *Pharm Biol*. 2015;53(12):1850-60.

[107] Mathew J, Gangadharan G, Kuruvilla KP, et al. Behavioral Deficit and Decreased GABA Receptor Functional Regulation in the Hippocampus of Epileptic Rats: Effect of Bacopa monnieri. *Neurochem Res*. 2011 Jan;36(1):7-16.

[108] Stough C, Lloyd J, Clarke J, et al. The chronic effects of an extract of Bacopa monniera (Brahmi) on cognitive function in healthy human subjects. *Psychopharmacology*. 2001;156:481-4.

[109] Dave UP, Dingankar SR, Saxena VS, et al. An open-label study to elucidate the effects of standardized Bacopa monnieri extract in the management of symptoms of attention-deficit hyperactivity disorder in children. *Adv Mind Body Med*. 2014 Spring;28(2):10-5.

[110] Kean JD, Downey LA, Sarris J, et al. Effects of Bacopa monnieri (CDRI 08®) in a population of males exhibiting inattention and hyperactivity aged 6 to 14 years: A randomized, double-blind, placebo-controlled trial. *Phytother Res*. 2022 Feb;36(2):996-1012.

[111] Crook T, Petrie W, Wells C, et al. Effects of phosphatidylserine in Alzheimer's disease. *Psychopharmacol Bull*. 1992;28:61-6.

[112] Kim HY, Akbar M, Lau A, et al. Inhibition of neuronal apoptosis by docosahexaenoic acid (22:6n-3). Role of phosphatidylserine in antiapoptotic effect. *J Biol Chem*. 2000;275:35215-23.

[113] Zanotti A, Valzelli L, Toffano G. Chronic phosphatidylserine treatment improves spatial memory and passive avoidance in aged rats. *Psychopharmacology (Berl)*. 1989;99:316-21.

[114] Spahis S, Vanasse M, Bélanger SA, et al. Lipid profile, fatty acid composition and pro- and anti-oxidant status in pediatric patients with attention-deficit/hyperactivity disorder. *Prostaglandins Leukot Essent Fat Acids*. 2008;79:47–53.

[115] Stanley JA, Kipp H, Greisenegger E, et al. Regionally specific alterations in membrane phospholipids in children with ADHD: An in vivo 31P spectroscopy study. *Psychiatry Res Neuroimaging*. 2006;148:217–221.

[116] Bruton A, Nauman J, Hanes D, et al. Phosphatidylserine for the Treatment of Pediatric Attention-Deficit/Hyperactivity Disorder: A Systematic Review and Meta-Analysis. *J Altern Complement Med*. 2021 Apr;27(4):312-322.

[117] Karanikas E, Daskalkis NP, Agorastos A. Oxidative Dysregulation in Early Life Stress and Posttraumatic Stress Disorder: A Comprehensive Review. *Brain Sci*. 2021 Jun;11(6):723.

[118] Lorenc-Koci E. Dysregulation of Glutathione Synthesis in Psychiatric Disorders. *Studies Psych Disorders*. 2014 Nov. Available at: https://link.springer.com/chapter/10.1007/978-1-4939-0440-2_14. Accessed January 7, 2023.

[119] Aruoma OI, Halliwell B, Hoey BM, et al. The antioxidant action of N-acetylcysteine: its reaction with hydrogen peroxide, hydroxyl radical, superoxide, and hypochlorous acid. *Free Radic Biol Med*. 1989;6:593–597

[120] Ghanizadeh A, Akhondzadeh S, Hormozi M, et al. Glutathione-related factors and oxidative stress in autism, a review. *Curr Med Chem*. 2012;19:4000–4005.

[121] Nikoo M, Radina H, Farokhina M, et al. N-Acetylcysteine as an Adjunctive Therapy to Risperidone for Treatment of Irritability in Autism: A Randomized, Double-Blind, Placebo-Controlled Clinical Trial of Efficacy and Safety. *Clin Neuropharm*. 2015 Jan/Feb;38(1):11-17.

[122] Ghanizadeh A, Moghimi-Sarani E. A randomized double blind placebo controlled clinical trial of N-Acetylcysteine added to risperidone for treating autistic disorders. *BMC Psychiatry*. 2013;13:196.

[123] Cui J, Shao L, Young LT, et al. Role of glutathione in neuroprotective effects of mood stabilizing drugs lithium and valproate. *Neuroscience*. 2007 Feb 23;144(4):1447-53.

[124] Prindle A, Liu J, Asally M, et al. Ion channels enable electrical communication in bacterial communities. *Nature*. 2015;527(7576):59-63.

[125] Forsythe P, Kunze WA, Bienenstock J. On communication between gut microbes and the brain. *Curr Opin Gastroenterol*. 2012 Nov;28(6):557-62.

[126] Fulling C, Dinan TG, Cryan JF. Gut Microbe to Brain Signaling: What Happens in Vagus... *Neuron*. 2019 Mar 20;101(6):998-1002.

[127] Bercik P, Denou E, Collins J, et al. The intestinal microbiota affect central levels of brain-derived neurotropic factor and behavior in mice. *Gastroenterology*. 2011;141:599-609,609.e1–609.e3

[128] Hata T, Asano Y, Yoshihara K, et al. Regulation of gut luminal serotonin by commensal microbiota in mice. *PloS One*. 2017 Jul 6;12(7):e0180745.

[129] Banskota S, Ghia JE, Khan WI. Serotonin in the gut: Blessing or a curse. *Biochimie*. 2019 Jun;161:56-64.

[130] Yano Jessica M, Yu K, Donaldson Gregory P, et al. Indigenous bacteria from the gut microbiota regulate host serotonin biosynthesis. *Cell*. 2015 Apr 9;161(2):264-76.

[131] Asano Y, Hiramoto T, Nishino R, et al. Critical role of gut microbiota in the production of biologically active, free catecholamines in the gut lumen of mice. *Am J Physiol Gastrointest Liver Physiol*. 2012 Dec 1;303(11):G1288-95.

[132] Hamamah S, Aghazarian A, Nazaryan A, et al. Role of Microbiota-Gut-Brain Axis in Regulating Dopaminergic Signaling. *Biomedicines*. 2022 Feb 13;10(2):436.

[133] McFarlin BK, Henning AL, Bowman EM, et al. Oral spore-based probiotic supplementation was associated with reduced incidence of post-prandial dietary endotoxin, triglycerides, and disease risk biomarkers. *World J Gastrointest Pathophysiol*. 2017, 8, 117–126.

[134] Lamprecht M, Bogner S, Schippinger G, et al. Probiotic supplementation affects markers of intestinal barrier, oxidation, and inflammation in trained men; a randomized, double-blinded, placebo-controlled trial. *J Int Soc Sports Nutr*. 2012 Sep 20;9(1):45.

[135] Wang B, Wu G, Zhou Z, et al. Glutamine and intestinal barrier function. *Amino Acids*. 2015 Oct;47(10):2143-54.

[136] Shu XL, Yu TT, Kang K, et al. Effects of glutamine on markers of intestinal inflammatory response and mucosal permeability in abdominal surgery patients: A meta-analysis. *Exp Ther Med*. 2016 Dec;12(6):3499-3506.

[137] Kim MH, Kim H. The Roles of Glutamine in the Intestine and Its Implication in Intestinal Diseases. *Int J Mol Sci*. 2017 May;18(5):1051.

[138] Achamrah N, Dechelotte P, Coeffier M. Glutamine and the regulation of intestinal permeability: from bench to bedside. *Curr Opin Clin Nutr Metab Care*. 2017 Jan;20(1):86-91.

[139] Santos J, Yang PC, Soderholm JD, et al. Role of mast cells in chronic stress induced colonic epithelial barrier dysfunction in the rat. *Gut*. 2001;48:630-6.

[140] Santos J, Benjamin M, Yang PC, et al. Chronic stress impairs rat growth and jejunal epithelial barrier function: role of mast cells. *Am J Physiol Gastrointest Liver Physiol*. 2000;278:G847–G854.

[141] Pearce FL, Befus AD, Bienstock J. Mucosal mast cells. III. Effect of quercetin and other flavonoids on antigen-induced histamine secretion from rat intestinal mast cells. *J Allergy Clin Immunol*. 1984 Jun;73(6):819-23.

[142] Weng Z, Zhang B, Asadi S, et al. Quercetin is more effective than cromolyn in blocking human mast cell cytokine release and inhibits contact dermatitis and photosensitivity in humans. *PLoS One*. 2012;7(3):e33805.

[143] Gao W, Zan Y, Wang ZJ, et al. Quercetin ameliorates paclitaxel-induced neuropathic pain by stabilizing mast cells, and subsequently blocking PKCε-dependent activation of TRPV1. *Acta Pharmacol Sin*. 2016 Sep;37(9):1166-77.

[144] Penissi AB, Rudolph MI, Piezzi RS. Role of mast cells in gastrointestinal mucosal defense. *Biocell*. 2003 Aug;27(2):163-72.

[145] Shi T, Bian X, Yao Z, et al. Quercetin improves gut dysbiosis in antibiotic-treated mice. *Food Funct*. 2020 Sep 23;11(9):8003-8013.

[146] Shigeshiro M, Tanabe S, Suzuki T. Dietary polyphenols modulate intestinal barrier defects and inflammation in a murine model of colitis. *J Funct Foods*. 2013 Apr;5(2):949-55.

[147] de Medina FS, Calvez J, Romero JA, et al. Effect of quercitrin on acute and chronic experimental colitis in the rat. *J Pharmacol Experiment Ther*. 1996;278(2):771-9.

[148] Suzuki T, Hara H. Quercetin enhances intestinal barrier function through the assembly of zonula [corrected] occludens-2, occludin, and claudin-1 and the expression of claudin-4 in Caco-2 cells. *J Nutr*. 2009 May;139(5):965-74.

[149] Amasheh M, Schlichter S, Amasheh S, et al. Quercetin enhances epithelial barrier function and increases claudin-4 expression in Caco-2 cells. *J Nutr*. 2008 Jun;138(6):1067-73.

[150] Nahrstedt A, Butterweck, V. Biologically active and other chemical constituents of the herb of Hypericum perforatum L. *Pharmacopsychiatry.* 1997;30 Suppl 2:129-134.

[151] Bhattacharya SK, Chakrabarti A, Chatterjee SS. Activity profiles of two hyperforin-containing hypericum extracts in behavioral models. *Pharmacopsychiatry.* 1998;31 Suppl 1:22-29.

[152] Demisch L, Holzl J, Gollnik B, et al. Identification of selective MAO-type-A inhibitors in Hypericum perforatum L. (Hyperforat). *Pharmacopsychiat.* 1989;22:194.

[153] Cott JM. In vitro receptor binding and enzyme inhibition by Hypericum perforatum extract. *Pharmacopsychiatry.* 1997;30 Suppl 2:108-112.

[154] Butterweck V, Winterhoff H, Merkenham M. St John's wort, hypericin, and imipramine: a comparative analysis of mRNA levels in brain areas involved in HPA axis control following short-term and long-term administration in normal and stressed rats. *Molecular Psych.* 2001;6:547–564.

[155] Kalb R, Trautmann-Sponsel RD, Kieser M. Efficacy and tolerability of hypericum extract WS 5572 versus placebo in mildly to moderately depressed patients: A randomized double-blind multicenter clinical trial. *Pharmacopsychiatry.* 2001;34(3):96-103.

[156] Linde K, Berner MM, Kriston L. St John's wort for major depression. *Cochrane Database Syst Rev.* 2008;(4):CD000448.

[157] Pakseresht S, Boustani H, Azemi ME, et al. Evaluation of pharmaceutical products of St. John's wort efficacy added on tricyclic antidepressants in treating major depressive disorder: a double blind randomized control trial. *Jundishapur J Nat Pharm Prod.* 2012;7(3):106-10.

[158] Asher GN, Gartlehner G, Gaynes BN, et al. Comparative Benefits and Harms of Complementary and Alternative Medicine Therapies for Initial Treatment of Major Depressive Disorder: Systematic Review and Meta-Analysis. *J Altern Complement Med.* 2017;23(12):907-19.

[159] Harrer G, Hubner WD, Podzuweit H. Effectiveness and tolerance of the hypericum extract LI 160 compared to maprotiline: a multicenter double-blind study. *J Geriatr Psychiatry Neurol.* 1994;7 Suppl 1:S24-S28.

[160] Harrer G, Schmidt U, Kuhn U, Biller A. Comparison of equivalence between the St. John's wort extract LoHyp-57 and fluoxetine. *Arzneimittelforschung.* 1999;49:289-96.

[161] Apaydin EA, Maher AR, Shanman R, et al. A systematic review of St. John's wort for major depressive disorder. *Syst Rev.* 2016;5(1):148.

[162] Hubner WD, Kirste T. Experience with St. John's Wort (Hypericum perforatum) in children under 12 years with symptoms of depression and psychovegetative disturbances. *Phytother Res.* 2001;15:367-70.

[163] Findling RL, McNamara NK, O'Riordan MA, et al. An open-label pilot study of St. John's wort in juvenile depression. *J Am Acad Child Adolesc Psychiatry.* 2003;42:908-914.

[164] Simeon J, Nixon MK, Milin R, et al. Open-label pilot study of St. John's wort in adolescent depression. *J Child Adolesc.Psychopharmacol.* 2005;15(2):293-301.

[165] Weber W, Vander Stoep A, McCarty RL, et al. Hypericum perforatum (St John's wort) for attention-deficit/hyperactivity disorder in children and adolescents: a randomized controlled trial. *JAMA.* 2008;299:2633-41.

[166] Lalousis PA, Schmaal L, Wood SJ, et al. Neurobiologically based stratification of recent onset depression and psychosis: Identification of two distinct transdiagnostic phenotypes. *Biol Psychiatry.* 2022 Oct 1;92(7):552-562.

[167] von Schacky C. Importance of EPA and DHA Blood Levels in Brain Structure and Function. *Nutrients.* 2021 Mar 25;13(4):1074.

[168] Titova OE, Sjorgen P, Brooks SJ, et al. Dietary intake of eicosapentaenoic and docosahexaenoic acids is linked to gray matter volume and cognitive function in elderly. *Age (Dordr).* 2013 Aug;35(4):1495–1505.

[169] Science Daily. Omega-3 Boosts Grey Matter, May Explain Improved Moods. Available at: https://www.sciencedaily.com/releases/2007/03/070307080827.htm. Accessed January 9, 2023.

[170] Chang JPC, Su KP, Mondelli V, et al. Omega-3 Polyunsaturated Fatty Acids in Youths with Attention Deficit Hyperactivity Disorder: a Systematic Review and Meta-Analysis of Clinical Trials and Biological Studies. *Neuropsychopharmacology.* 2018 Feb;43(3):534-545.

[171] Lefevre-Arbogast S, Dhana K, Aggarwal NT, et al. Vitamin D Intake and Brain Cortical Thickness in Community-Dwelling Overweight Older Adults: A Cross-Sectional Study. *J Nutr.* 2021 Sep 4;151(9):2760-2767.

[172] Walhovd KB, Storsve AB, Westlye LT, et al. Blood markers of fatty acids and vitamin D, cardiovascular measures, body mass index, and physical activity relate to longitudinal cortical thinning in normal aging. *Neurobiol Aging.* 2014;35:1055–64.

[173] Ibrahim F, Halttunen T, Tahvonen R, et al. Probiotic bacteria as potential detoxification tools: assessing their heavy metal binding isotherms. *Can J Microbiol.* 2006 Sep;52(9):877-85.

[174] Bisanz JE, Enos MK, Mwanga JR, et al. Randomized Open-Label Pilot Study of the Influence of Probiotics and the Gut Microbiome on Toxic Metal Levels in Tanzanian Pregnant Women and School Children. *mBio.* 2014 Oct 7;5(5):e01580-14.

[175] Tian F, Zhai Q, Zhao J, et al. Lactobacillus plantarum CCFM8661 alleviates lead toxicity in mice. *Biol Trace Elem Res.* 2012 Dec;150(1-3):264-71.

[176] Kullisaar T, Songisepp E, Aunapuu M, et al. Complete glutathione system in probiotic Lactobacillus fermentum ME-3. *Prikl Biokhim Mikrobiol.* 2010 Sep-Oct;46(5):527-31.

[177] Lahlou M. Essential oils and fragrance constituents: bioactivity and mechanism of action. *Flav Frag J.* 2004 Mar/Apr;19(2):159-165.

[178] Buchbauer G, Jirovetz L. Aromatherapy – use of fragrances and essential oils as medicaments. *Flav Frag J.* 1994 1994 Sep/Oct;9(5):217-22.

[179] Costa R, Machado J, Abreu C. Evaluation of Analgesic Properties of Piper Nigrum Essential Oil: a Randomized, Double-Blind, Placebo-Controlled Study. *World J Tradit Chinese Med.* 2016;2(2):60-64.

[180] Komori T, Fujiwara R, Tanida M, et al. Potential antidepressant effects of lemon odor in rats. *Eur Neuropsychopharmacol.* 1995;5:477–480.

[181] Choi MS, Choi BS, Kim SH, et al. Essential Oils from the Medicinal Herbs Upregulate Dopamine Transporter in Rat Pheochromocytoma Cells. *J Med Food.* 2015 Oct;18(10):1112-20.

[182] Johnson SA. Beating ADHD Naturally. Scott A Johnson Professional Writing Services, LLC: Orem, UT, 2016.

[183] Santos NAG, Martins NM, Sisti FM, et al. The cannabinoid beta-caryophyllene (BCP) induces neuritogenesis in PC12 cells by a cannabinoid-receptor-independent mechanism. *Chem Biol Interact.* 2017 Jan 5;261:86-95.

[184] Johnson SA, Rodriguez D, Allred K. A Systematic Review of Essential Oils and the Endocannabinoid System: A Connection Worthy of Further Exploration. *Evid Based Complement Alternat Med.* 2020 May 15;2020:8035301.

[185] Martins LB, Tibaes JRB, Sanches M, et al. Nutrition-based interventions for mood disorders. *Expert Rev Neurother.* 2021 Mar;21(3):303-315.

[186] Croll PH, Voortman T, Ikram MA, et al. Better diet quality relates to larger brain tissue volumes: The Rotterdam Study. *Neurology.* 2018 Jun 12;90(24):e2166-e2173.

[187] Kokubun K, Yamakawa Y. Association Between Food Patterns and Gray Matter Volume. *Front Hum Neurosci.* 2019 Oct;13:384.

[188] Bauer ME, Teixeira AL. Inflammation in psychiatric disorders: what comes first? *Ann N Y Acad Sci.* 2019 Feb;1437(1):57-67.

[189] Van Lent DM, Gokingco H, Short MI, et al. Higher Dietary Inflammatory Index scores are associated with brain MRI markers of brain aging: Results from the Framingham Heart Study Offspring cohort. *Alzheimers Dement.* 2022 May 6;10.1002/alz.12685.

[190] Mikkelsen K, Stojanovska L, Polenakovic M, et al. Exercise and mental health. *Maturitas*. 2017 Dec;106:48-56.

[191] Tempesta D, Salfi F, de Gennaro L, et al. The impact of five nights of sleep restriction on emotional reactivity. *J Sleep Res*. 2020 Oct;29(5):e13022.

INDEX

pesticides, 17

phosphatidylserine, 48-49

phospholipid, 48

physical activity, 3, 71-72

physiological, 12, 57

processed foods, 18, 71

poultry, 15

probiotics, 23, 52-55, 65-66

Prozac, 37

psychophysiological, 52

psychotherapy, 31, 36

psyllium, 22

PTSD, 12, 30

Q

quercetin, 23, 56, 57

quetiapine (Seroquel), 41

R

reactive hypoglycemia, 17-18

reactive oxygen species, 49, 50

relationships, 9, 10, 14, 74

reversal learning, 25-26

risperidone (Risperdal), 39-40, 44, 50

Ritalin, 34

S

salicylates, 17

salmon, 15, 63

sardines, 63

sauna, 24

school, 7, 10, 12, 14, 74

seeds, 15, 20

self-medicating, 13

senna, 22-23

sennosides, 22-23

sensory avoiding, 28

sensory processing, 27-28

sensory seeking, 28

sensory sensitivity, 28

serotonin, 14, 15, 21, 29, 37, 38, 39, 46, 48, 52, 53, 55, 57, 59, 66, 71, 72

serotonin transporter gene, 14, 29

severe mood dysregulation disorder, 11, 39

shellfish, 17

siblings, 9, 10, 32

sleep, 24, 35, 36, 38, 40, 43, 46, 67, 72-73

SNRIs, 36-38, 43

soy, 17, 20, 71

spinach, 15

SSRIs, 37-38

stimulants (stimulant medications), 33, 34-35, 39, 43, 46, 48, 58, 59, 66, 67

stimuli, 25, 26, 27, 28

stress, 14, 15, 17, 18, 21, 29, 46, 48, 52, 55, 57, 58, 71

St. John's wort, 57-59

STIs, 14

stress axis, 14

substance abuse, 13, 14

sugar, 17-18, 70
suicide, 15, 30, 37, 38, 42

T

temper, 9, 10, 11, 12, 39, 42
thioridazine (Mellaril, Melleril), 40-41
threat, 27, 33, 57
trauma, 13, 14, 49, 57
tryptophan, 15
tuna, 15, 63
turmeric, 23

U

urine testing, 22

V

vagus nerve, 52
valproate sodium, 42, 51
vegetables, 15, 18, 19, 56, 69, 70, 71
venlafaxine (Effexor), 36
violence/violent, 14, 15, 19, 21, 36, 37, 39
vitamin C, 15
vitamin D, 15, 62-63

W

water, 19, 20, 21, 23, 63
watermelon, 15
whole grains, 15, 69, 70

www.ingramcontent.com/pod-product-compliance
Lightning Source LLC
Chambersburg PA
CBHW070614220526
45467CB00003B/1430